MENDING MINDS

A Series of Books in Psychology

Editors:
Richard C. Atkinson
Gardner Lindzey
Richard F. Thompson

MENDING MINDS

■■■

*A Guide to the New Psychiatry of Depression,
Anxiety, and Other Serious Mental Disorders*

Leonard L. Heston, M.D.
Professor of Psychiatry
The University of Washington

Director
The Washington Institute for
Mental Illness Training and Research

W. H. Freeman and Company
New York

Library of Congress Cataloging-in-Publication Data

Heston, Leonard L.
Mending minds : a guide to the new psychiatry of depression, anxiety, and other mental
disorders / by Leonard L. Heston.
p.   cm.
Includes bibliographical references and index.
ISBN 0-7167-2158-9. — ISBN 0-7167-2167-8 (pbk.)
1. Psychiatry—Popular works. 2. Depression, Mental—Popular works. 3. Anxiety—Popular
works. 4. Mental illness. I. Title.
[DNLM: 1. Anxiety Disorders. 2. Depressive Disorder. 3. Personality Disorders. 4. Psychotic
Disorders. 5. Schizophrenia. 6. Substance Use Disorders. WM 170 H588m]
RC460.H47, 1991
616.85'27—dc20
DNLM/DLC
for Library of Congress   91-25061
                                                                               CIP

1 2 3 4 5 6 7 8 9 0   VB   9 9 8 7 6 5 4 3 2

Contents

□ □ □

MENDING MINDS

Introduction

□ □ □

A QUIET revolution has been occurring in psychiatry. Treatments for mental disorders have greatly improved, bringing important practical benefits to mentally ill persons and their families. Although "cures" have not been attained and may never be, today's treatments make it possible for many of those affected by mental illness to manage their condition effectively, or even largely disregard it, in their daily lives.

The fact that so many people become mentally ill magnifies the importance of these medical advances. Nearly one person in five will develop a major psychiatric illness over the course of his or her lifetime. Providing basic information to these persons, their families, and their friends is a central aim of this book. This knowledge is important because, today, psychiatric treatment increasingly involves both patients and their families as full participating partners in the ongoing management of the illness. Those concerned need to know the facts about the diagnosis, treatment, and prognosis of mental illness.

A further aim of this book is to introduce the broader public to the striking advances that have taken place in modern behavioral science and to psychiatry's prominent place in these advances. Medicine has long appreciated that the royal road to understanding normality is through study of the abnormal. The subject matter of psychiatry is abnormal human behavior. Though not all human behavior is understandable from the perspective of psychiatric medicine and behavioral science, much more is now known than most people realize. Moreover, outlines of further advances are emerging. The developing knowledge and power of psychiatric medicine will directly affect not only ill persons and their families but also our institutions—government, schools, and courts, as well as medicine itself. The ramifications will extend into all corners of our society.

I well remember my decision in the early 1960s to specialize in psychiatry. I had chosen medicine because I was interested in human behavior. This interest led me to study the brain. My first choice was neurosurgery, but the operations I participated in as an intern, which consisted mainly of sucking away diseased brain tissue with an aspirator, seemed far removed from behavior. Neurology would have been my next choice, except that neurologists were preoccupied with reflexes and tended to ignore thought and emotion.

That left psychiatry. At the time, I felt that psychiatry was not particularly advanced as a medical science and feared that I would be so dissatisfied that I would regret having changed specialties. It was a difficult decision, but today I know my choice was right for me. As it turned out, any of the three choices would ultimately have been a good one: All of medicine has changed, including neurosurgery and neurology. But psychiatrists, especially, sense that they have leapfrogged over other specialties and are set to move all of medicine ahead.

This enhancement of psychiatrists' self-esteem is recent. Although psychiatrists are physicians—fully trained medical doctors—they were often only partly accepted by the medical profession. This stance goes back to the Middle Ages, when the mentally ill were regarded as "possessed" and so were thought to be the responsibility of religious authorities, not medicine. It was not until the late nineteenth century that medicine at last began to accept psychiatric patients. Then, support for their treatment became the responsibility of governments because psychiatric patients were too ill and ill too long to be able to pay for their own medical care. The result was the state hospital system. (Tuberculosis and leprosy were the other important diseases given over to state medicine.) State hospitals dominated psychiatric treatment until the advent of psychoanalysis after World War II.

Psychoanalysis was practiced in offices, not hospitals, and it served a population that could pay its own way handsomely. Treatment was based on Sigmund Freud's theory of personality development. Illness was thought to result from psychic trauma that caused repression of associated drives, feelings, and memories. Healing entailed becoming consciously aware of these unconscious mental processes and, most important, re-experiencing the emotions associated with the original trauma. But the rush of enthusiasm for psychoanalysis that swept over American medicine was soon followed by disillusionment. Its promise of effective treatment was not kept, especially for the more severe illnesses. Moreover, psychoanalysis failed as a science because it did not develop testable hypotheses, the foundation of scientific investigation.

Despite these failures, modern psychiatry owes a debt to psychoanalysis. The humane treatment of mentally ill patients, the recognition that we are unaware of some of our motivations, and even the optimism about the eventual discovery of effective treatments are important legacies. Today, however, psychiatry's focus has shifted from abstract descriptions of postulated mental processes to the actual study of the brain as a biologic tissue. That change in emphasis has been the source of the major advances in understanding and treating mental illness that are the subject of this book, and it has demonstrated once and for all that the methods of general medicine are equally applicable to psychiatry. These methods definitely include the "art" of medicine: the willingness to listen to patients with sensitivity, patience, and caring, individual attention and to make understandable to each patient the major features of the illness and the options that exist for treating it. Perhaps because of the influence of psychoanalysis, psychiatrists are particularly adept in these skills and in medical centers are usually the teachers of the needed techniques.

This book is concerned with conditions that are widely acknowledged to be mental diseases, as well as with other conditions, such as "personality disorders," that are associated with problematic behavior but have not been proved to be diseases. Some subjects will not be covered. A few diseases are too rare or esoteric to be included here, and childhood mental illness is a subject that needs its own, separate book. Nor will the reader find elaborate theorizing, guru-isms, blaming of mothers for unhappiness, backbiting among contending schools, or prescriptions for instant mental health. Such topics were a product of pre-science and are no longer a part of what most psychiatrists actually do.

Psychiatric illness is known by the changes it produces in broad functional areas, such as thought, emotion, perception, and behavior. Because these changes are interrelated, most psychiatric illnesses produce some change in more than one or two of these areas. Specific illnesses are defined in terms of the particular combination of changes, the order in which the changes appeared, and which contributes most to the disability. General medicine also defines disease in terms of what combinations of bodily events occur (such as pain, fever, and swelling) and how they are ordered in time and severity. Accordingly, this book is organized into six parts, each of which focuses on a major category of psychiatric change and the illnesses in which that change is the salient feature. A seventh part discusses current views of the causes of the problematic changes and what the future is likely to bring. Practical steps that mentally ill persons, and those close to them, can take to help manage the illness are highlighted, as, for example, in the section titled "If you are depressed." Other special sections, such as "How Drugs Work in the Brain" and "The Insanity Defense," are devoted to important scientific or societal topics. These are areas wherein psychiatry contributes to medical knowledge or interacts with the social establishment.

Case histories (largely those of some of my own patients, with details changed so that identification is not possible) are used to illustrate the different illnesses. Descriptions of actual people with actual illnesses best convey medical information and make it memorable. These anonymous individuals are the heroes and heroines of this book. They also represent all the other patients to whom I am indebted for the warm emotional rewards and constant intellectual challenges that have enriched my professional life. I hope they find, in this book, some small payment on the debt I owe.

1

MOOD
...

Mood is our prevailing emotional tone—how we feel—over several hours or days; in contrast, *affect* is how we feel from moment to moment. Mood is therefore a rough average of affects experienced over time. The illnesses of mood are marked by its extreme high, mania, and by its extreme low, depression. The distinction between mood and affect is critical to understanding mania and depression, and to help students in behavior science understand and remember it early in their studies, they are given this saying to ponder: "Mood is to affect as climate is to weather."

Both mood and affect are subjective; that is, they are known only to the person experiencing them. In this respect, they are like pain. This means that another's mood or affect must be somehow communicated if we are to learn what feelings he or she is experiencing. Usually others tell us about their mood or affect through a rich vocabulary: happy, sad, blue, low, excited, turned on, top of the world, and so on. Most of our common greetings ("How have you been?") are inquiries or statements about each other's mood or affect. We also estimate other people's affect without being told by observing their *psychomotor responses*—facial expressions, gestures, and tone of voice. We may say someone looks "down in the mouth" or "like the cat that swallowed the canary." These psychomotor responses are partly involuntary, innate responses. Infants who are born blind develop psychomotor expressions of their feelings identical to those of seeing persons, despite their having no model for the behavior. Although a good actor or a "poker face" may sometimes deceive us, most people's psychomotor responses accurately reflect their feelings.

Affect and psychomotor responses can be viewed as the results of parallel physiologic processes. Our brains are organized such that information from our senses is distributed to several processing channels. One of these channels has two main outputs: (1) internal feelings and (2) commands to muscles that result in psychomotor responses. Feelings reflect the subjective value that we place on the events in our lives, rewarding or punishing us, whereas psychomotor responses communicate these feelings to the externaL world.

Although affect is evoked mainly by our external world, we can also create imaginary worlds that, by simulating sensory input, produce real affect. In normal life we do this through daydreaming and fantasy. In most mental illness, however, our affective responses to both external and internal stimuli are distorted.

The intensity and direction of affect are influenced by our overall mood, and likewise, a series of positive or negative affects can combine to influence mood. A compliment from one's boss increases the likelihood that one will experience a happy mood over the next few days. Unhappy events can produce the opposite result. The affects we experience, then, interact with our prevailing mood. And the same event may strike us differently, depending on whether our mood is mildly depressed or elated. All of us experience these variations in affect regularly.

Illness of mood is different from these common ups and downs. It is depression or elation far more extreme than normal, everyday moods, and it cannot be explained by the influence of external events. Understanding illnesses of mood requires that we achieve a new understanding of mood itself—one different from that which suffices in ordinary life. Otherwise, we may fall prey to the same sort of errors in thinking about the causes of mood disorders that have plagued humans since they started thinking about themselves. For example, if we are depressed, ordinary reasoning tempts us to assume that un-happy events must have caused the condition and that what we need is corrective happy experiences. In illness, this assumption is faulty on both counts: Unhappy events do not cause depressive disease, and happy events cannot cure it. Rather, the mood change is produced by internal physiologic processes that are largely (though not complete-ly) independent of external events.

The first chapter in this section covers depressive illness. The topics range from diagnostic methods to the treatments available. The following chapter describes bipolar (manic-depressive) illness and its treatment.

Chapter

1

Depression
□ □ □

❏ *John*

John and his wife lived in a suburb of a major city, where he taught biology and chemistry in the high school from which both had graduated. They had raised two children, both adapting reasonably well to adult life. At age 51, John considered himself a typical family man: happy in his work, financially secure, stable in his marriage and his community. However, that summer his illness began.

One night he awoke at 3 A.M., hours before his usual time, gripped by feelings of hopelessness and dread. Gradually, the unformed dread became focused on the coming day and a routine teachers' meeting scheduled for the purpose of preparing for the new school year. In other years this had been a pleasant reunion, this morning it loomed as a terrifying ordeal. Agitated and apprehensive, John paced through the house for the next three hours. Finally, he made coffee and then began to feel a little better. That day he found the meeting enjoyable after all.

Two nights later a similar episode occurred. And this time, before it ended, he was gripped by an intense, smothering pain that seemed to envelop his heart. John had a sense that death was near. Even so, this episode also passed. That day he painted a room in his house and that night enjoyed a movie with his wife.

During the next week John's mood worsened. He continued to awaken in the early morning to feelings of a pervasive melancholy—his "great black hole." No matter where his thoughts turned, he found unrelieved gloom. Pride in his accomplishments was replaced by despair over what he now saw as a life of failure after failure: in college, in the navy, as teacher, as lover and husband. Everything he was today, everything he had, seemed worthless. His future seemed hopeless, too horrid to think about. Sometimes he knew that his pessimism was exaggerated, but though he tried hard to do so, he could not change his outlook. Focusing his thoughts elsewhere did not help; neither did reading nor watching television—after a few seconds his morbid ruminations returned. Often he wept silently.

The mornings continued to be the worst time of the day, but his afternoons also became troubled. He spent most of the day pacing. When he found that alcohol provided a little relief, he began drinking beer. Soon he was drinking a six-pack every afternoon and often drank another three or four bottles during the evening. He rarely bathed or brushed his teeth. Although he never really rested, John was unable to sleep through the night. He continued to rise early and mope around the house. By evening he usually felt better, but the combination of beer and lack of sleep made him sluggish. Bed came early, and once there, he had no trouble getting to sleep, though it was a troubled sleep that ended too soon.

His wife tried reason. "How can you say you've failed your students?" she would say. "Just look at your two 'Best Teacher' awards. And other teachers elected you their delegate to the state education convention." Friends and their clergyman advised her to "get him out of himself...start him on healthy activities." She worked hard. She prepared his favorite meals, which he ate out of habit but without appetite or pleasure. She arranged outings such as bowling and picnics, and she invited friends to their home. To be sure, John did sometimes perk up and seem almost his old self. But those times grew less and less frequent. Even sex held little interest for him. Although his wife often took the initiative, he was sometimes impotent and sometimes too preoccupied with his worthlessness—to which sexual failure was an incidental addition.

Nearly three weeks dragged by, and John, desperate for relief, began planning suicide. Although he was sure that his chest pains, which returned from time to time, were due to some fatal illness, but he found waiting for a natural death intolerable. Despite deeply felt religious prohibitions, he decided on suicide by carbon monoxide poisoning. He checked his will and insurance policies, located a suitable hose to attach to the exhaust of his automobile, and wrote a short note to his wife. He was ready, except for one loose end. Thirty years before, he had used his mustering-out pay from the Navy to make a down payment on 40 acres of land, long since paid for, which he now rented to a farmer. Thinking about simplifying his estate and getting cash for his widow, he began trying to sell the land. Although he was willing to sell at distress prices, completing a sale was complex and would take time. That delay saved his life.

One night John had a pang of chest pain that was worse than usual, and his wife insisted that they go to the emergency room of a nearby hospital. After an electrocardiogram and other laboratory examinations of his heart proved normal, the emergency room doctor suspected depression or some other brain disease and called a consulting psychiatrist. On the basis of descriptions provided by John and his wife, the psychiatrist agreed that depression was the most probable diagnosis, and an initial treatment plan was developed. John was given a prescription for a standard antidepressant drug (amitriptyline, or Elavil). He was to take one tablet (50 milligrams) each evening until his appointment with the psychiatrist. That conventional start-up dose was much too small for adequate treatment, but to John's great surprise—for he was sure nothing could help him—and to his wife's great relief, he began to sleep through the night. This one change seemed to make everything else notably better.

Despite this encouraging change, John did not really want to see a psychiatrist. Neither he nor his wife thought he was "crazy." Also, they had known a woman who had seen a psychiatrist twice a week for several years, after which she was more "mixed up" than when she had started treatment. So they canceled John's appointment, and for several days he limped along on his small dose of antidepressant.

During this period the school year began. John, an experienced and competent teacher, managed his classes fairly well. Yet his continued preoccupation with his miserable failures and hopeless future made it impossible, much of the time, to concentrate. He was also intolerably anxious. After his classes, but while still in the school building, he continued his afternoon drinking. The drinking and the other changes in him became so obvious that the principal of the school called his wife and insisted on a medical examination. In response to this pressure, John finally made another appointment with a psychiatrist.

After examining him, the psychiatrist prescribed higher doses of the antidepressant drug and instructed that the dose be increased fairly rapidly to a maximum determined by John's responses. He also prescribed an antianxiety drug to be used sparingly (instead of alcohol) in the afternoons, and John was instructed to take sick leave for the following week and to make no business decisions. In particular, he could not sell his land, and to be sure that he did not, his wife was advised to hold the title. He was to return in one week.

John found several things about that first visit surprising. The systematic questioning seemed to touch firmly on each feature of his illness, as though everything he had been going through—the early morning awakenings, the wish to die, and all the rest—were part of a well-known pattern. Also, the psychiatrist was interested in his family. John had forgotten, until he was questioned, that on two or three occasions during his childhood, his mother had been away from home for weeks at a time with "breakdowns" and that one of her brothers had killed himself. His wife, too, was shocked when she learned just how far her husband's plans for suicide had progressed.

Over the next few days, with increased doses of the antidepressant, John improved dramatically. After a week, at a dose of

150 milligrams, he felt nearly normal. The drug caused him to feel a bit weak, and his mouth was uncomfortably dry, but his mood had become as optimistic as ever. He used only two tablets of the antianxiety drug and stopped drinking entirely. After he had taken the antidepressant drug for two months, the dose was gradually reduced to 50 milligrams. However, at this level, John's sleep again became disturbed, so the dose was increased to 100 milligrams.

Now, four years after the diagnosis, John continues to take small doses of the antidepressant drug, usually 50 milligrams a day. On three occasions, his sleep disturbance has threatened to return, but briefly increasing the dose to 150 milligrams restored normal sleep. All attempts to stop the medication entirely have failed, because without it John's mood again becomes depressed—not a common outcome, but far from unknown and not alarming. His weakness has not continued, but dryness of the mouth has remained a problem. Perhaps because of the drug, he has tended to gain weight. All in all, John thinks that the benefits of the drug far outweigh these relatively minor problems. Today his life goes on in its former happy patterns. He remembers his "great black hole" very well, but he hardly ever thinks about it.

■ Diagnosis, Prognosis, and Dis-ease ■

An organized and logical approach to an illness such as John's requires making a *diagnosis* and formulating a *prognosis*. A diagnosis is an hypothesis about the cause of distress. An examining doctor attempts to match all the information available about a patient's distress to a *syndrome*—a cluster of signs and symptoms of disordered function that tend to occur together and are usually related anatomically, physiologically, or chemically. For example, cramping, upper-right abdominal pain after meals, jaundice, and clay-colored stools are elements of a syndrome that suggests obstruction of the bile ducts by gallstones. It is often possible to go on to identify what specific disease is causing a syndrome (for example, a blood test might implicate a disease interfering with cholesterol metabolism as a contributing cause of gallstones), but most psychiatric illnesses are known only at the syndrome level. The fit of signs and symptoms to syndromes is seldom perfect. It is a "preponderance of the evidence" that supports diagnostic conclusions, and it is not necessary that every finding that characterizes a syndrome be present for diagnosis to be made. Too, an individual may present signs or symptoms that are not usually included in the syndrome.

Careful diagnosis enables medical specialists to predict what is likely to happen to an individual who exhibits specific signs and symptoms of illness. This prediction—a prognosis—is based on what happened, on average, to persons who once exhibited the same syndrome. Though not perfect when applied to individuals, predictions based on diagnosis are fairly accurate. Diagnoses make possible rational estimates of what the available treatments are likely to accomplish, compared to one another and compared to no treatment at all. This link among diagnosis, prognosis, and treatment forms the scientific basis of all modern medicine.

Prognoses vary in accuracy according to the amount of information available on a particular syndrome or disease. Estimating the course for a case of chicken pox can be done quite precisely; for major depression, less so; and for cancer of the thyroid gland, less yet. Evidence has been collected over decades to support useful prognoses for psychiatric diseases. These predictions are sometimes more accurate, but perhaps more often are less accurate, than medicine's general average, but they are always far ahead of random, uninformed guessing. Of course, no two people experience exactly the same outcome from a given disease. Recognizing factors unique to every ill person that modify the course and outcome of disease, and making judicious allowance for them, are the essence of the art of medicine. These skills are as applicable to major depression as to any other illness.

Psychiatric diagnoses are different from most other medical diagnoses in one important respect. Many manifestations of psychiatric disease—even the most incapacitating—have features that also appear in normal persons. Like John, most of us have at some time become depressed and anxious. However, John's depression was clearly beyond the range of normal experience, and that is the key. Illness is present when our sense of well-being, our ease, is disturbed enough to become *dis-ease,* and the disturbance is seen as something apart from our normal life. At root, all definitions of illness depend on those distinctions.

The concept of dis-ease will be important as we consider various psychiatric conditions. The discomfort produced by dis-ease is also the basis of some unfortunate misunderstandings. Most of us recognize discomforts such as anxiety and depression as a normal part of life that we tolerate reasonably well most of the time. We may wonder, then, whether the dis-ease felt by people just a bit less ill than John is really more than the transient woes inflicted on us by the ordinary ups and downs of life. Maybe such people expect unreasonable comfort. Maybe, like spoiled, demanding children, they refuse to tolerate the dis-ease that the rest of us muddle through nearly every day. Why can't they just "tough it out"?

These are not illogical questions, but the answer is that the majority of people who have received psychiatric diagnoses experience distress much more intensely than others do. No one puts forth their full effort all of the time. At times, everyone can tolerate more distress before they complain or seek sympathy or take a day off from work. But overall, we all—including people with psychiatric diseases—put forth close to our best efforts most of the time.

■■■

Diagnosis: Major Depression

John's diagnosis was major depression. This is a common disease: Some 12 to 18 percent of the population will experience it sometime during their lives. For those who reach late middle age, the estimate is near 30 percent. For unknown reasons, females are affected about twice as often as males. Onset may occur at any age.

Major depression is a cycling disease; once established, it tends to get better over time and then to return again. Anyone who has had one episode is therefore at increased risk for subsequent episodes, which may appear at fairly regular intervals. An average of 12 months for a complete cycle is a figure often cited. But a cycle can last for years.

Signs and Symptoms

The accompanying table gives the approximate percentage of people who experience the main signs or symptoms of major depression. Such a tabulation is a useful summary, but it cannot possibly convey a sense of what John lived through. Depressed mood, the first entry in the table, permeates all aspects of life. John's major depression meant that the values he placed on his possessions, personal relationships, past accomplishments, and future prospects were distorted by a strong negative bias proportional to the depth of the depression. (John's would be considered moderately severe.) Interest in everyday activities evaporates because no pleasure accompanies them. Of course, the future to offers only pain. Memories of the past consist only of failure heaped upon failure through life. Guilt for past sins must be massive to justify the terrible punishment they are feeling, so depressed persons are painfully preoccupied with guilt. Even if suicide is punished by damnation, that may not be too high a price to pay to escape the unbearable hell of the present.

John was spared only one of the major features of depression, weight change. Sufferers usually lose weight, but sometimes they gain. A decrease of 10 to 20 percent of body weight is not uncommon and is a useful diagnostic flag. Few illnesses are associated with weight loss of that magnitude; it is a sign of major illness, very commonly depression.

John had a typical depressive sleep disturbance, getting to sleep at his usual bedtimes but awakening much earlier than usual. For depressed persons, those early morning hours are the worst time of the day, a common time for suicide.

Another entry in the table, diurnal variation in mood, warrants further comment. Depressed people often experience changes in affect through the day. Typically, they feel most depressed in the morning hours and then improve as the day goes on; evenings may even be pleasant. This can lead to serious misunderstandings on the part of physicians, other professionals, and family members who are not aware

SIGNS AND SYMPTOMS OF MAJOR DEPRESSION

Sign or Symptom[1]	Percent Manifesting
Depressed Mood	100
Loss of interest	92
Excessive feelings of guilt	54
Irritability	37
Hopelessness about the future	78
Wishes for death	66
Plans for suicide	33
Weight Change	85
Loss	70
Gain	15
Sleep Disturbance	82
Insomnia (waking too early)	65
Oversleeping	17
Others	80
Overactivity (anxiety)	45
Slowed thinking and/or movement	23
Excessive fatigue	60
Poor concentration	74
Neglect of hygiene	46
Variation in mood during the day	57
Constipation	44

[1] A *sign*, such as temperature, blood pressure, or serum cholesterol level, is observable. A *symptom*, such as pain or mood, is not observable.

of the distinction between mood and affect. Many an exasperated spouse has said something like, "Last night you had a grand old time playing pinochle with your cronies, but now this morning I can't get you to stop moaning long enough to eat breakfast." Such changes over a short time may make it appear that the depressed affect is voluntary and that mood could be improved by just a little change in attitude, a little bit of effort. Not so. The most profoundly depressed mood may be interrupted by brief periods of normal or even elevated affect. Why nature tends strongly to place the more normal periods later in the day is unknown, but the fact that it does provides a useful guide both for diagnosing depression and for interaction with depressed persons.

Prognosis

Without treatment, the outcome of an episode of major depression is not just months of intense suffering. Afflicted persons also have about a 30 percent greater risk of death than members of the general population of the same age. About half of this increased risk is due to suicide (see Box 1). The balance is due to a variety of conditions, such as heart disease and infections. The suicide risk is understandable, but just why depressed persons should be at higher risk of death from other causes is not fully understood. Several factors probably contribute, among them self-medication with alcohol or other drugs, and neglect of personal hygiene and diet.

Treatment radically changes the course of major depression. By the time all available treatments have been used, normal mood returns in about 90 percent of cases. Usually, as in John's case, only one course of treatment is necessary, and that approach stimulates a prompt response. The cyclic nature of major depression means that many affected persons improve even when nothing is done. But even allowing for this, there can be no doubt that today's treatments, which are described later in this chapter, are a huge improvement over letting the illness take its natural course. They are effective and safe—a victory for humankind over a most painful disease.

Other Types of Depression

Major depression is the most common of the severe mood-associated illnesses that psychiatrists treat. There are, however, other types of serious depression that have different causes, which often means they present different problems and require different treatments.

Secondary Depression

Depression is often a secondary effect of other illnesses. Indeed, depressed mood is commonly associated with illness, and though it rarely approaches the intensity seen in major depression, it can be quite serious. Cancer and heart disease, for example, are life-threatening, often painful conditions that sap vitality. Here depressed mood is understandable, and though there is considerable variability, the depth of the depression can be roughly related to the seriousness of the illness.

Other psychiatric illnesses are also associated with a secondary depression, no doubt for the same reasons: Feeling ill and being disabled by a psychiatric disorder *is* depressing. Complications arise, though, because now two disorders are affecting mental state: the original condition and the secondary depression associated with it.

Depression also commonly exaggerates other, unrelated problems. For example, John's inconsequential chest pain seemed to him a sign of catastrophic illness. Depression may also exaggerate psychiatric symptoms: A mild tendency to excessive anxiety may escalate into a disabling condition. It may be difficult for a psychiatrist to discern whether depression is causing a minor physical problem or personality trait to worsen so that it appears to be a diagnosable illness in its own right or whether a major illness is producing a secondary depression. One helpful clue is the age of the patient when the illness began, because illnesses have characteristic ages of onset. For example, an anxiety disorder beginning in middle age would lead the psychiatrist to suspect depression. As primary illnesses, anxiety disorders typically begin much earlier in life, often in adolescence.

Depression as a Side Effect of Drugs

Many drugs used in general medicine can produce depression as a side effect. Drugs used to treat high blood pressure (hypertension) are especially notable. The most common offenders are preparations containing reserpine (such as Serpasil, Unipress, Hydropres); propranolol (Inderal); methyldopa (Aldoclor, Aldomet, Aldoril); and clonidine (Catapres). The hormones cortisone, estrogen, and progesterone often produce changes in mental state, including depression. Levodopa (Sinemet, Lardopa), which is used to treat Parkinson's disease, has frequently been associated with depression. These by no means exhaust the list, and it is only good medical practice to suspect drugs in any case of depression—or in any other change in mental state.

Grief

Bereavement, the medical term for grief, is regarded as a normal response to the loss of a loved one, usually through death. During bereavement, the full range of depressive signs and symptoms can be observed. Studies of groups of bereaved persons have found that depressed mood usually worsens during the first few weeks following bereavement, and during this time the use of alcohol and other sedative drugs tends to increase. Mood improves after the first month and by the third or fourth month, the major signs of depression disappear and those affected report feeling much better. By six months, normal mood has largely been restored, and by one year, recovery is effectively complete. However, flashes of depression triggered by reminders of the loved one often persist beyond the first year, but they occur less frequently and are usually less intense. Statistically, bereavement does not result in an overall increase in hospitalizations for any reason, including psychiatric, or in an increase in suicides. However, hidden in the figures may be a slight increase in deaths related to alcohol abuse or suicide among bereaved men over age 55. These deaths tend to occur in men who were alcoholic before their bereavement.

Though painful and distressing, bereavement generally is tolerated reasonably well and is associated with little or no lasting disability. If major illness of any sort develops during the period of bereavement and persists, its onset is most likely to be coincidental. Severely depressed mood persisting more than six months beyond bereavement is treated as major depression.

Postpartum (Puerperal) Depression

Pregnancy poses no increased risk for psychiatric illness. Indeed, it is a happy fact that most psychiatric illnesses spontaneously improve during pregnancy. However, the postpartum period—the period immediately after childbirth—is another matter. During this period, and tapering off over the next several weeks, there is an increased risk for a major illness, especially depression. Postpartum depression is quite distinct from the "new-baby blues," a minor disturbance of mood so common after childbirth that it is regarded as normal. A postpartum depression has all the features of a major depression, often an extraordinarily severe one, and it may begin abruptly. Its cause is unknown but is thought to be related to hormonal changes associated with childbirth. The risk is increased for women who have had previous depressions or whose family members have illnesses of mood.

Postpartum depression occurs in only a small proportion of women with newborn babies (about 1 to 2 per 1000 births), but it is especially important to recognize, because one common feature is fear of taking care of the infant. An affected woman has a gloomy assessment of her ability to care for the child physically, feels unworthy of love from the child or anyone else, and is preoccupied with guilt and failure. Too often, what follows is actual inability to care for the infant and outright rejection of it. This affliction is hard for new fathers to understand, much less sympathize with, and it may destroy the expected joys of a happy birth, the making of a family, and the natural bond between mother and infant. What should be the happiest of events develops potential for tragedy. But if the illness is recognized, treatment is usually gratifyingly effective.

Treatment

Nearly all depressions can be treated successfully. Treatment restores a normal mood in about 90 percent of persons with a major depression. Moreover, responsiveness usually returns to ordinary ranges; successfully treated persons respond to events in the same way they did before developing major depression. The same is true of nearly all women who experience postpartum depression.

Drugs are the first of the treatments of depression that we will describe. Drugs are endemic to our society and they are also crucial to understanding other psychiatric conditions. Before going on, an overview of drugs and the brain will be helpful.

Box 1   Suicide and Mental Illness

Suicide is the eighth leading cause of death among Americans. In the early 1980s about 30,000 suicides were registered on death certificates each year, but this is certainly an underestimate, because equivocal evidence of suicidal intent and pressure from families lead physicians and medical examiners to minimize reported suicide.

Searches for the causes of suicide lead directly to psychiatric illness. Studies of the immediate past history of persons who have succeeded in committing suicide reveal that 90 to 95 percent had chronic psychiatric illness. Another 3 to 4 percent had major nonpsychiatric illness, such as cancer or multiple sclerosis. Less than 1 percent had no medical diagnosis. The psychiatric illnesses consisted of mood disorders, schizophrenia, and chemical dependency—all treatable diseases. Looked at another way (that is, starting with diagnostic groups instead of successful suicides), 25 to 30 percent of persons with mood disorder, 10 to 20 percent of those with schizophrenia, and 15 to 25 percent of those who are dependent on chemicals eventually kill themselves. Suicide is clearly the major risk factor associated with psychiatric illness. It follows that one of the chief responsibilities of psychiatrists is to estimate their patients' risk for suicide. The stakes are high and the evidence is never conclusive. In practice, the ten-

■ Drugs and the Brain ■

Barely 30 years ago, effective drug treatments began to percolate into psychiatric practice. They have since created a revolution by making it possible to control the disabling signs and symptoms of previously untreatable psychiatric

dency is to err on the conservative side simply because death cannot be undone.

In addition to psychiatric illness, factors that increase the risk of suicide include being over 45, being male, being Caucasian, being unmarried, living alone, and not working. Psychiatrists have found a few other clues that help sharpen predictions. A complete and workable plan for suicide is one. John had this. Attempting to provide ample cash and an easily managed estate, as John did, is another. Making a will and attempting to buy insurance are other alarm signals. These are helpful clues, but there is no way to be certain whether a patient will make a suicide attempt. A psychiatrist is never without several patients at high risk for suicide, and a few always succeed in killing themselves.

Preventing suicide requires getting adequate treatment for persons who are depressed or at risk for other reasons. This may include forced hospitalization and (sometimes) physical restraint within the hospital. At times there is no other way. One further note: Suicide prevention centers, despite extraordinary and selfless efforts by largely volunteer staffs, have not succeeded in lowering the rates of completed suicide in their localities. It appears that most people who call these centers are just people who want to talk. Apparently, individuals genuinely at risk for suicide do not tend to avail themselves of suicide prevention centers or "hot lines."

disorders. Hospitals emptied (sometimes too rapidly), but for a large proportion of those discharged, drugs made a reasonably productive and rewarding life possible. Because of these effective treatments, many were spared the terrible interruptions of life that mental illness once imposed. All of our research confirms that drug treatment of mental illness has been enormously beneficial. Drug treatment is not a perfect answer—far from it—but many of those who decry the pharmacologic revolution in psychiatry forget how bad things were before these drugs were available.

Pharmacology also created revolutionary changes in theories about the origins of human behavior and mental illness. Drugs are chemicals. They are capable of interaction only with other chemicals, yet they influence profoundly such central attributes of human mental activity as mood and thinking. This understanding, together with advances in the field of genetics, undercut theories based in one way or another on the separation of body and mind, discrediting mid-century theories of mental illness. As a practical example of this process, if pharmacology was mentioned at all in mid-century psychiatry coursework, it was clearly regarded as an unworthy, somehow contaminated treatment option. Today, pharmacology is a core subject.

The pharmacologic revolution is by no means over. New drugs, most of them based on sophisticated neurochemical theory, are constantly being tested. Some pass muster and become an accepted part of medical practice, where they continue to spell improvements in the lot of ill persons. But there may be a darker side. It is not unreasonable to fear *Brave New World* outcomes (passivity, sapping of initiative, the use of drugs to control rather than cure) from brain pharmacology. Will it one day be possible to so finely modulate brain activity with drugs that some combination of perfect contentment with just enough variation to keep mental life interesting can be artificially maintained? If so, individuals could attain their personal nirvana while never leaving their couches. Our experience with drug abuse does not reassure us on this point. Will brain pharmacology be used by despots to make docile workers and fierce soldiers? Most of the belligerents in World War II gave amphetamines (speed) to elite fighting units. Such hazards should not be forgotten, but surely the promise of effective medical treatment far outweighs the dangers. In any event, societal and individual choices involving drugs that affect brain function will contribute to shaping our future world.

Drugs work by altering the brain's chemistry. Nerve cells, or neurons, communicate with one another through chemicals emitted by one neuron that affect an immediately adjacent neuron. These chemicals are called *neurotransmitters*; a dozen are known to be important in the brain, and there are probably at least twice that many. The place at which a neurotransmitter is released by one neuron and received by another is called a *synapse*—a small space where two nerve cells are very close together but do not touch. At a synapse the transmitting neuron, known as the presynaptic neuron, emits a little cloud of neurotransmitter to the receiving, or postsynaptic, neuron.

A typical neuron receives messages—some stimulating, some inhibiting—from thousands of other neurons, each at a different synapse. When the balance of stimulating messages that one neuron receives passes a threshold, the neuron "fires," stimulating the neurons to which it transmits.

The messages exchanged by neurons constitute the information processing of the brain. The information itself is everything we know or feel; it is our knowledge of the world around us and the status of our bodies; it is our memories, our thoughts, our impulses, our mood, our loves and hates, our humanness, and (through reflexes established during evolution) responses "learned" during our animal history.

The important features of neurotransmission are depicted in the figures on the following page, which we will refer to as a general model throughout this book, especially with respect to the actions of drugs.

The process of neurotransmission is influenced by drugs in several ways. Here are some examples.

• Many neurotransmitters are stored in small packets—*synaptic vesicles*—located within nerve cells near a synapse. Some drugs shortcut the normal communication process by releasing neurotransmitters from their vesicles, thereby stimulating receiving neurons.

• To transmit its message, a neurotransmitter emitted into the synaptic cleft fits into receptors on the surface of the receiving neuron. Neurotransmitter and receptor molecules have a precise lock-and-key relationship based on their physical shapes

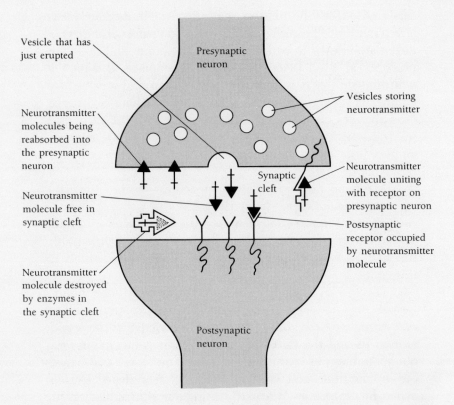

Vesicle that has just erupted

Presynaptic neuron

Vesicles storing neurotransmitter

Neurotransmitter molecules being reabsorbed into the presynaptic neuron

Synaptic cleft

Neurotransmitter molecule uniting with receptor on presynaptic neuron

Neurotransmitter molecule free in synaptic cleft

Postsynaptic receptor occupied by neurotransmitter molecule

Neurotransmitter molecule destroyed by enzymes in the synaptic cleft

Postsynaptic neuron

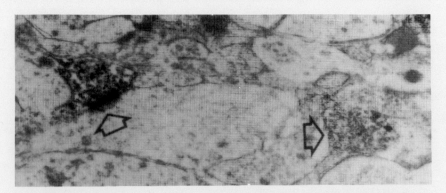

Electron microscopic image of a neuron with two synapses indicated by the open arrows. These synapses have been stained to show the neurotransmitter serotonin as black granules.

and electro-chemical affinities. Normally, only one chemical, the neurotransmitter used at that synapse, can fit the shape of the receiving cell's receptors and stimulate it. This stimulus is then passed through the receptor protein into the receiving neuron, where it activates that cell's machinery. Many drugs and poisons work by mimicking the physical properties of a neurotransmitter well enough to stimulate its receptor. Others occupy receptors without stimulating them, thus blocking the neurotransmitter and preventing it from acting.

• *Autoreceptors* tell transmitting neurons how much neurotransmitter traffic is flowing within the synapse. In response, the transmitting neuron may change the rate of production or the availability of neurotransmitter. At least one drug, cocaine, acts by blocking autoreceptors for specific neurotransmitters, thus freeing transmitting neurons from inhibition and increasing the production of transmitter.

• Once released, a neurotransmitter cannot normally remain in the synaptic cleft, because its signal must be turned off. Of the thousands of neurotransmitter molecules emitted, some are destroyed by enzymes within the synaptic cleft. But biologic systems are thrifty and efficient, so most molecules are reabsorbed by the transmitting neuron, to be stored again in vesicles and used time after time. Some drugs prevent or slow the destruction of neurotransmitter within the synaptic cleft; others prevent reabsorption. Either mechanism results in greater stimulation of the receiving neuron.

■■■

Antidepressant Drugs

Several drugs have antidepressant properties, but by far the the most effective and most often used fall into two major groups. These consist of the *tricyclics* and the *MAOIs*; MAOI stands for "monoamine oxidase inhibitor."

Tricyclic Antidepressants

Since about 1960, the "first line of defense" in the treatment for depression has been a category of drugs known as tricyclic antidepressants (so called because of their three-ringed chemical structure). Tricyclic antidepressants inhibit the reabsorption into the transmitting neuron of two neurotransmitters, norepinephrine and serotonin. This makes the two neurotransmitter molecules available to receptors for a longer time, and receiving neurons get additional stimulation. Just how this improves mood is unknown, but that these transmitters are important to mood is supported by the action of reserpine, a drug that produces depression as a side effect. When given over a period of time, reserpine depletes the brain's stores of both norepinephrine and serotonin.

The different tricyclic drugs are classified according to their relative sedating or alerting properties. The accompanying table lists the major tricyclic drugs and their most important clinical characteristics. In deciding which such drug to prescribe, psychiatrists are guided most by the sedating properties of the drug. Some people with depression tend to be agitated. If so, a more sedating drug is used. Depression may also be associated with lethargy, in which case a more alerting drug is appropriate.

Tricyclic drugs are usually started at about one-third the estimated final dose, which is then increased over four or five days. The

TRICYCLIC ANTIDEPRESSANTS RANKED FROM 0 TO 4 BY INCREASING SEDATIVE ACTION

Trade Name(s)	Chemical Name	Sedating Effect
Aventyl, Pamelor	Nortriptyline	0
Ludiomil	Maprotiline	1
Norpramin	Desipramine	1
Tofranil, Janimine	Imipramine	1
Ascendin	Norpramine	2
Desyrel	Trazodone	2
Surmontil	Trimipramine	2
Vivactil	Protriptyline	2
Elavil, Endep	Amitriptyline	3
Adapin, Sinequan	Doxepin	4

entire dose is often taken an hour or so before bedtime. Although it is often said that these drugs may take up to three weeks to be effective, this statement is misleading. Improvement is nearly always obvious within a few days if a drug is effective. Then several days may be required before the drug exerts its maximum effect on mood. Often re-establishment of a normal sleep pattern is the first sign of improvement, as it was in John's case. The outcome of successful treatment is complete normalization—a modern miracle of pharmacologic science.

Current practice is to maintain the effective dose for three to four weeks and then reduce it by one-third. The lower dose is maintained for two to three months and then slowly reduced to zero. (All drugs that act on the brain should be withdrawn gradually.) If mood worsens at any time during the withdrawal process, increasing the dose will restore the previous state within a couple of days. Ordinarily, the order in which signs of illness appear remains constant. For example, if sleep disturbance was a first sign of illness, it will usually be so again if a relapse develops as a drug is withdrawn. It will also be a reliable herald of future episodes, even years later. Learning what symptoms mark the early stages of illness *for a particular person* is a most important goal of the educational process necessary in all medical treatment.

The tricyclic antidepressants have so far proved remarkably safe. The most common significant side effect of their ordinary use is faintness (*syncope*), which results from a fall in blood pressure. When this occurs, it is not serious, except in elderly people who may be injured in falls. This is one reason why a starting dose for elderly people should be much smaller (perhaps 10 percent of the estimated final dose), and increases should be smaller and more widely spaced. If syncope occurs, it usually appears when the patient is moving from a reclining to a more upright position. The only way to prevent this is to rise slowly, giving the body plenty of time to adjust the blood pressure to the change. If a severe problem persists, adjustments may have to be made in the dose of drug, or the drug preparation may have to be changed, or support hose may be needed to help blood return to the heart from the legs.

Almost always, the tricyclic antidepressants produce excessive fatigue during the first period of their use. A fine tremor of the extremities, blurred vision, impotence, difficulty voiding urine, and constipation are also fairly common early in the course of treatment. After about two weeks, these unwanted effects—as well as syncope—tend to decrease and then disappear.

This is not true of two other undesirable effects, dry mouth and weight gain, which usually remain. Dry mouth is caused by a decrease in moistening saliva, a result of the direct effect of tricyclic antidepressants on the autonomic nervous system, which controls involuntary responses such as salivation. If dry mouth occurs, as it nearly always does, it is likely to remain through the course of treatment. Lemon lozenges or, better, a mouthrinse consisting of about 20 parts glycerine to 1 part lemon oil may be helpful. Both glycerine and lemon oil can be purchased in most drugstores. The mechanism by which tricyclics produce weight gain is unknown, but it often includes a craving for carbohydrates. Weight gain is not a problem for everyone, but for those bothered by it, gaining several pounds over a short period can be a problem.

A more serious side effect of the tricyclics (happily it is a rare one) is that they may aggravate certain heart conditions. Tricyclic drugs prolong the electrochemical impulses that normally cause coordinated contraction of the heart muscle. This is inconsequential for normal hearts, and tricyclics are, in fact, used to treat certain kinds of heart disease (such as first-degree heart block). But there are heart disturbances—mainly bundle branch block—that tricyclics can dangerously worsen. If heart disease is present, tricyclics may have to be used cautiously or not at all. Doctors are alert to the possible consequences for the heart of tricyclic treatment. Patients aware of any heart problem should be sure that their doctor knows about it. If there is any doubt, an electrocardiogram should be done before, and sometimes during, a course of treatment.

Despite all these cautions, the tricyclics are among medicine's safest drugs. Many persons with a chronic, long-lasting depression take antidepressants for decades, or even a lifetime, with no adverse effects and can be reasonably confident of the drugs' safety and continued effectiveness.

A special consideration in the use of all drugs is their potential for harming unborn children. Tricyclics have not, so far, been shown to harm the unborn. Nevertheless, as a general principle of sound medical practice, all drugs should be avoided during pregnancy, especially during the first three months. As we have noted, major affective illness seldom occurs during pregnancy, so few pregnant women seek treatment for it. Because drugs of all kinds, including antidepressants, are secreted in milk, nursing mothers can give a substantial dose to their infants. Thus, although there is no proven risk to the infants, most nursing mothers are wise to avoid antidepressants as well as other drugs.

Monoamine Oxidase Inhibitors

Monoamine oxidase is an enzyme that is normally present in all tissues, including the brain, where it is active within cells and within synaptic clefts. It breaks down the neurotransmitters serotonin and norepinephrine. Since an MAOI drug prevents monoamine oxidase from destroying those neurotransmitters, their concentration increases, causing increased stimulation of their postsynaptic neurons.

As has been the case for nearly all other drugs, the usefulness of MAOIs was discovered by accident. An early MAOI preparation was used to treat tuberculosis; later, it was noted that the tubercular patients became uncharacteristically active and happy. Building on this clue, therapists tried the drug as a treatment for depression. By the mid-1960s, it and several of its near relatives became standard treatments for depression. MAOIs are often the first choice of treatment for secondary or atypical depressions, and they are used for major depression as well if the patient's response to tricyclics is not satisfactory.

MAOI drugs characteristically produce immediate stimulation, with increased muscle activity, decreased fatigue, and greater social spontaneity. Mood is elevated for the first few days of treatment, but this tends not to persist, and there may be a few days of partial relapse into depression before mood becomes normal again. It may take 10 to 14 days at maximum dosage for the treatment to stabilize at its most effective point.

The unwanted effects of the MAOI drugs are similar to those of the tricyclics, but they are more variable. Usually blood pressure falls, which may cause fainting. For reasons not well understood, persons predisposed to migraine headaches often find that MAOIs make that problem worse. There is no information about use in pregnancy, but again, common sense strongly suggests that pregnant women avoid any drug that is not absolutely essential.

A rare but serious side effect of MAOI use is a sharp, severe rise in blood pressure called a hypertensive crisis. This can occur because MAOIs interfere with the normal breakdown of tyramine, a chemical that, through an indirect mechanism, causes blood pressure to rise rapidly. The danger sign is usually a severe headache. This has an abrupt onset, usually within half an hour of eating tyramine-rich food, and it tends to start at the back of the head. Vomiting, chest pain, and restlessness are commonly associated with the headache. Although the attack is usually short-lived, subsiding over the course of an hour and ending soon thereafter, it is an unmistakable sign of trouble. A specific antidote (phentolamine) is available in hospital emergency rooms.

Because of the risk of hypertensive crisis, persons taking MAOI drugs *must avoid* foods containing large concentrations of tyramine. The most dangerous are those in which protein degeneration has begun; such as aged cheeses, sweetbreads, unpasteurized red wine, yeast extracts, and smoked meats. When MAOIs are prescribed, the doctor should supply the patient with a detailed lists of foods to avoid. (Most pharmacies can also supply such a list.)

Some drugs can produce serious problems when taken with MAOIs. The most common of these are nasal decongestants and cough medicines that contain ephedrine, phenylephrine, or phenylpropanolamine. But the most dangerous drugs—potentially lethal, in fact—are the "street" stimulants amphetamine and cocaine. The danger of hypertensive crisis persists for about two weeks after the last dose of an MAOI, because it takes that long for the body to restore monoamine oxidase to its normal level.

Just describing the side effects of drugs can lead to unwarranted fear of their use, and this has been the case with the MAOIs. After it became known that MAOIs could sometimes produce hypertensive crisis, the drugs were not often prescribed. Serious complications are rare, however, and the dietary restrictions are not too onerous. MAOIs are powerful agents that demand respect, but that same power is what makes them effective in treating serious disease.

Other Antidepressant Drugs

During the past five years several new antidepressant drugs have been introduced. Whereas older antidepressants increase the action of three main neurotransmitters (norepinephrine, serotonin, and dopamine), the newer drugs generally have relatively pure actions on only one. For example, one group selectively inhibits the reuptake of serotonin into nerve cells. The first of these drugs to be marketed, fluoxetine (Prozac), has so far proved effective in some depressions that were previously resistant to treatment. However, doubts have begun to cloud Prozac's prospects. A side effect of this class of drugs is weight loss, and it appears that the drug is being prescribed increasingly for weight reduction. Some persons taking the drug have developed dangerously agitated conditions, and it is possible that the drug is more of a stimulant than a true antidepressant. It takes some time before practical experience with a new drug permits comprehensive definition and evaluation of its effects; Prozac is currently undergoing this process. Meanwhile, it is proving to be an effective drug for some depressed persons, and it has been the impetus for intensive pharmacologic research that is yielding other new products. Optimism is certainly warranted.

Electroconvulsive Therapy

Abbreviated ECT and also known as *electroshock* and *shock treatment,* electroconvlusive therapy is one of the most dramatically effective and safest of all medical treatments. Yet it has become as controversial as any treatment in the history of medicine. When described, it can sound barbaric, and no one knows just why it is effective. But dozens of careful studies have shown that it is a highly effective, and often life-saving, treatment.

Electroshock therapy was discovered by accident. There are several stories about how this happened, but a credible one is this: In the mid-1930s, a physician observed that the mood of depressed epileptic patients improved after an epileptic seizure. This led to the therapeutic induction of seizures in other patients. Two main methods were tried, injection of convulsant drugs and electroshock. The latter was found to be safer and more effective. The first results reported from hospitals around the world seemed miraculous. After a few treatments, patients who had been ill for years became normal. Excitement and optimism ruled psychiatry as never before.

During the 1930s and 1940s hospitals were full, and there were no effective treatments for any psychiatric disease. Then suddenly, thanks to ECT, miraculous cures were effected daily. To anyone familiar with the history of medicine, what happened next will be no surprise. ECT was tried on any patient for whom no other treatment was available; in psychiatric hospitals this meant virtually every patient. It just might work, and besides, it was the only hope. (In medicine, too, if your only tool is a hammer, every fastener looks like a nail.) Nonpsychiatric medicine offers many examples of grossly overused treatments, both effective and ineffective: penicillin, cortisone, hysterectomy, removal of teeth (to cure "foci of infection"), to name a few. In the case of ECT, the huge crush of desperately ill patients seemed to leave no time to work out sophisticated techniques for administering the treatment. Tens of thousands of patients were treated. Although the treatment itself produced no pain because unconsciousness immediately followed the first passage of electricity, the convulsion was violent. Three or four strong aides held patients down. Muscle and bone injuries were common.

Apart from injuries due to the convulsion, the only common side effect was a retrograde amnesia: Memory was lost for the period just before the treatment. In a young, healthy brain, the loss was a matter of a few minutes; an older or impaired brain might lose an hour or so. The time period for which memory was lost increased with each treatment; within very rough limits, the second treatment obliterated about twice as much as the first, and so on. There was also a period of confusion following treatment that sometimes persisted for several minutes—longer in older persons. The periods of true amnesia for events before treatment merged with this period of confusion. By the end of a usual course of treatment, an older person might have only patchy memories of a hospital stay and, because of this loss of connections, might become quite confused. Much (though not all) of the lost memory was restored over the next few days, with consequent reversal of confusion.

Memories established before the first treatment were preserved intact. Also, carefully designed tests of intellectual ability given before and after courses of ECT, including tests of ability to learn newly presented material, failed to demonstrate permanent loss of any mental ability. Indeed, test scores often improved, presumably because of improvement in the mental illness for which the treatment was administered.

Psychiatrists remain troubled, however, by occasional patients who insist that their treatment with ECT caused a permanent disturbance in memory. Sometimes this conviction can be attributed to the negative thinking that results from a recurrence of mental illness such as depression. But complaints of other persons are not so easily dismissed. Although no one can fully account for such cases, my experience suggests the following explanation. As noted above, ECT causes gaps in memory for periods immediately before each treatment. These gaps may be long or short, but they are always there. Most people find this side effect tolerable. They accept the gap and do not dwell on it. But occasionally a patient finds the loss extremely disquieting and becomes painfully preoccupied with trying to reconstruct the missing pieces. These may be the people who come to think of themselves as damaged by ECT.

In the decades since the development of ECT, the treatment has been greatly improved. First, ECT is now used mainly for major depressions and sometimes for secondary depressions. Other uses have been largely dropped over time. Second, it is given while the patient is under general anesthesia produced by a rapidly acting barbiturate, with muscles made completely flaccid by an injected drug, succinylcholine. This prevents convulsive movements. As a result, patients no longer have to be held down, and bone and muscle injuries do not occur. An anesthesiologist administers these drugs and gives oxygen during the period of paralysis.

Another refinement involves placement of the electrodes. In past practice, an electrode was placed on each temple so that the current passed through the frontal areas of the brain. It is now clear that stimulation of only one side of the brain, the nondominant side (usually the right side), produces less memory disturbance. Electrodes are therefore placed on the right forehead and either at the vertex of the head (the crown) or behind the right ear. This practice is now preferred in many localities.

Electroshock entails no more risk than minor surgery. In our university hospital, we have not had even a minor complication for as long as anyone can remember; the same is true across the country. ECT is effective and safe not only for persons without complicating disease but also for persons with severe brain or heart disease. It is also the safest treatment for use during pregnancy.

■ *If You Are Considering ECT*

If ECT is recommended by your doctor, and if you agree to the treatment, you must sign a permission form. There may be some preliminary examinations, such as x-rays of the spine, and an electrocardiogram, but as the safety of modern procedures has grown more evident, these precautions have come to be required less frequently. The night before each treatment, you must not eat or drink after midnight. This is a routine precaution taken before any anesthesia is administered. The next morning, you will walk to the treatment room, climb onto a wheeled stretcher, and lie down. Usually the treatment team, whom you will get to know, will converse and joke with you while the anesthesiologist starts an intravenous injection in your arm and injects a rapidly acting barbiturate (often Brevitol). You will feel a very pleasant sleep beginning—and nothing else. After your sleep begins, a powerful muscle relaxant, succinylcholine (Anectine), will be injected, and the anesthesiologist will begin administering oxygen.

Meanwhile, the psychiatrist will have set up the ECT equipment. Often this includes electrocardiographic and electroencephalographic leads attached to your chest and scalp in order to monitor your heart and brain activity. The machine will be set to deliver a precise current for a precise length of time. A common initial setting is 0.6 amperes for one and a half seconds. About 90 seconds after the succinylcholine is given, electrodes will be placed on your head, a button will be pushed, and the current will pass between the electrodes. Because the current passes through facial muscles, they will contract, but there is no other movement unless too little succinylcholine has been given. If so, the movements will be so weak as to be inconsequential, but more succinylcholine may be given next time. The psychiatrist will read the electroencephalogram to be sure that your brain is showing seizure activity for a sufficient time—ideally, at least 30 seconds. Rarely, the seizure is too short, and the psychiatrist may decide to administer another stimulus. After another minute or two the paralysis will begin to lift, and after 5 minutes you will begin to awaken. By this time all the medical equipment will have been disconnected and you will be in a recovery room.

You will feel groggy for about 10 minutes, but then you will feel well enough to leave and you will probably want to eat. After an hour, except possibly for a headache (due to the anesthesia, not to ECT itself), you will be entirely recovered. Even after one treatment, you may well find your depression improved. Usually, perceived improvement is greatest immediately after each treatment. But then the depression will slowly return until your next treatment. Usually treatments are given every other day through the work week. After each one, your improvement will last longer than it did after the previous treatment. After three or four treatments you will probably know that you are going to recover.

Six to eight treatments, on average, are given for depression. Some psychiatrists give a prescribed number, say eight. Others gauge the number given by the response. My own rule of thumb is this: Treat until the patient's mood is normal just before the next scheduled treatment. Then end the course of treatment with that one. ECT given as the only treatment for depression is successful with around 90 percent of those who receive it.

Bright-Light Therapy

Over the past six years, researchers have treated a special type of depression with intensive exposure to bright light. This kind of depression is highly seasonal; it typically begins in October and November and persists until March or April. For this reason it is known as seasonal affective disorder, or SAD (one of medicine's better acronyms). Mood is depressed, but unlike what is found in most depressions, weight is usually gained, not lost, and sleep is excessive—often 15 or 16 hours a day. The added sleep tends to occur during the morning. The effect of environmental light on the brain and its role in controlling daily cycles of hormone release were known to researchers, so it seemed reasonable that these atypical depressions might result from faulty adaptation to the decreased light of winter.

The treatment consists of nothing more than exposure to two hours of bright light in either the morning or evening. The light source is intense—several times brighter than a brightly lit office. This new treatment is still far from having been proved effective. But it may turn out to be the treatment of choice for certain highly selected depressed persons.

Psychotherapy

In psychiatry as in every health profession, verbal interactions among professionals, patients, and families have crucial initial objectives. The responsible professional must provide conditions that promote free communication and must discover and break down the barriers that might hinder gathering the information necessary to understanding the experiences of the ill person and the place of the illness in the affected person's particular social milieu. The next objective is to make all concerned understand the diagnosis, prognosis, and treatment options as thoroughly as possible. Next, every effort must be made to minimize the disruption of life, and especially the distortion of personal relationships, produced by the disease. Depending on their training and experience, various practioners use different methods to attain these objectives. Each develops an individual style. No matter what the practitioner's theoretical persuasion, if he or she is well trained and is a sensitive human being, the predisposition will not interfere with practical adjustment to the specific needs of an ill person.

Psychotherapy has those same objectives in treating depression, but with two important modifications. The potential for suicide must be estimated, and the wisdom of interventions involving personal relationships must be weighed against the depth of the depression. In depression as severe as John's, intensive inquiry and efforts to modify interpersonal relationships should usually be limited to simple reassurances. Unwise interventions can make matters worse, because depression distorts judgment and biases memory in negative directions. Attempts to address problems that may not really exist, in an effort to help a person who cannot in any case believe that a solution is possible, not only waste time, but can produce lasting scars within families. The most sensitive practitioners explain this to those involved and defer that type of exploration until the depression is better, when it may well turn out not to be needed. In contrast, milder depressions may well benefit from interpersonal explorations guided by a skilled psychotherapist. Making the needed distinctions along the continuum from "severe" to "mild" requires finely honed professional judgment.

This type of intervention is known as supportive psychotherapy. It may range from the exchange of a few sentences to several hours of professional contact with a psychiatrist, psychologist, nurse, or social worker. The aim of these professionals is to minimize the disability the illness produces by encouraging of constructive actions, while at the same time being reasonably sympathetic to the distress the patient feels. This is a delicate task. Illness of any sort, if it lasts for even a little while, produces reverberations throughout the patient's whole social network—family, job, friendships. It makes little difference whether the condition is depression, an orthopedic injury, or a heart attack. Not only are the social consequences inevitable, but too often they interfere with recovery. Constructive change often requires the direction and support of an objective professional.

Family education is an important aspect of supportive therapy. It is the job of professionals to instruct patients and their families systematically in the nature of the illness and in how best to cope with it. Everyone concerned should understand the signs and symptoms of the illness involved. It is especially important to know the early signs of an improving or worsening condition, the wanted and unwanted effects of drugs, the effects environmental features are likely to have, and the legacy of the disease itself over time. Patients and families should become as well versed as any professional in their particular illness in all its unique features. The instruction in these matters can be done individually, in groups, in family meetings, or through some combination of these settings. It can be done by a physician, a psychologist, a nurse, or a social worker—whatever professional is most knowledgeable and best positioned.

Cognitive therapy is a special technique of psychotherapy. It was developed over the last decade and shows promise for treating depressions, especially some of the milder ones. Largely practiced by psychologists, cognitive psychotherapy seems closely related to an earlier approach called rational emotive psychotherapy. The treatment consists of a systematic examination of attitudes, especially attitudes toward self. It seeks to change, by rational examination, self-defeating responses that have become habitual. This reasonable, commonsense approach is being actively explored as a therapeutic tool, either alone or in combination with drugs and general supportive management.

■ *If You Are Depressed*

Taking note of the following points may help. First, it is no doubt difficult for you to believe that you can possibly be helped. Depression obliterates hope, including hope of recovery. Yet modern treatments usually completely reverse depression. So try to acknowledge the possibility that you will get better. Patience may be required, however, because several treatments are available, and their effectiveness varies from case to case. Doctors have become quite good at picking out the treatment that is most likely to work for a particular person, but sometimes they miss and then must try an alternative. Don't give up.

Second, most people describe depression as breaking over them in waves. (Others use stronger terms, such as avalanche.) A sign that treatment is succeeding is that the waves break less often and tend to recede faster. But even though they come less frequently, the waves will remain strong until they stop coming altogether. This is important to remember, because it contradicts our common-sense understanding of the healing process. Unlike the healing of cuts and scrapes, in which every day brings visible progress and the injury does not get worse, recovery from depression (and most other psychiatric disorders) does not proceed steadily in a straight line. Expecting similar steady progress while recovering—but all the while experiencing new waves of depression as bad as any known before—can be terribly discouraging. It will help you a little to expect such waves, to brace yourself against them, and to know that this is the usual course of resolution. Focus on the increasing intervals between the waves.

■ If Someone Close to You Is Depressed

John's wife made most of the well-meant errors committed by family members who misunderstand the nature of major depression. She tried to cheer John up and to kid or jolt him out of his depression—which is what we all try to do when dealing with a minor mood shift. Such tactics have little effect on major depression, but there are several helpful things that can be done:

• It is especially important to recognize depressive illness by the major clues it gives. Early wakening, weight loss, and loss of interest in previously pleasurable activities are useful clues.

• Insist on a professional evaluation. Remember that depressed people are negative about everything, including the likelihood of successful treatment. You must take charge. Be as forceful as you need to be to get the job done.

• Try to prevent the depressed person from making any major decisions. Depression distorts judgment, which predisposes one to errors that may be hard to reverse.

• Neither try to argue an affected person out of depressive distortions nor agree with her or him. Do accept as a fact that this person finds life unbearably awful. It helps just to be understood.

• Try to make sure that the affected person gets adequate nutrition. Ensuring adequate fluid intake is the first priority and is usually sufficient.

• Guard against suicide. You can't eliminate all opportunities, but do the best you can. At least get firearms, ammunition, and poisons (including prescription drugs) out of the home. Remember that the early morning hours are often especially difficult.

2

Bipolar Disorder

Manic-Depressive Illness

□ □ □

❑ *Karen*

Karen was 26 years old when she began her residency in pediatrics at a major teaching hospital. Despite a boyish appearance that made her seem too young and playful for serious work in medicine, she knew she would succeed. She had an engaging, happy personality that, coupled with her assertive personal style, projected an air of confident, assured youth. She felt exhilarated as she moved into her apartment in a building where the hospital housed some of its residents.

The next week her duties began. A few days later, she was well acquainted with her new colleagues and her first patients. These patients were children treated with bone marrow transplants; most had cancer, all were terribly ill. More than half of them would die, never leaving the hospital. Sick and vulnerable children can be depressing to work around, but Karen was more deeply affected than most of her colleagues. She developed a depression much like the one John experienced over the first half-dozen days of his illness. She had little appetite, had trouble sleeping past 3 A.M., and felt discouraged and fatigued.

But soon her mood changed dramatically. One morning she awoke and, for no reason at all, felt wonderfully exhilarated. The day flew by as Karen moved effortlessly through her routines. That night, content and glowingly optimistic—in a "pink spell," as she later described it—she sang and danced about her apartment holding a pillow until dawn.

During the next few weeks she was tireless, feeling every pain of her small patients and tending to each one with skill and compassion. Talkative, friendly, outgoing, and so unflaggingly cheerful that she was nicknamed "happy doc," Karen endeared herself to the patients and the staff of her ward.

One day, about two months into her residency, she happened to notice an advertisement in a local medical newsletter. A union was offering to award a group of doctors a contract to conduct comprehensive examinations of its membership. A total of 1857 men were to have physical and screening laboratory examinations. Depending on what these examinations revealed, some of these men would then need such other tests as electrocardiograms or examinations by various specialized physicians. Karen quickly estimated that each initial examination would take the average physician about an hour. With mounting excitement, she calculated that the examinations would constitute a year's work for one physician. Why, she thought, not her?

That night Karen couldn't sleep. She sang and danced around her apartment, and she thought about what the contract required. The next morning she named herself the Nerak Clinic (Nerak is Karen spelled backward), got herself some letterhead stationery, and submitted a bid to do the examinations for $99.98 each. She chose this amount because she anticipated competitive bids at $100, but, in fact, the only other bid was over $200. Karen was soon awarded the contract.

The precise sequence of events over the next six weeks is unclear, but the outcome became a local legend. While managing her duties as a resident at the same pace as before, Karen completed the examinations she had contracted to do and submitted the results to the union. Even though they thought they were dealing with a group of doctors, union officials were astonished that the terms of the contract had been so quickly fulfilled. They made a thorough audit of the work and found it to be complete and accurate. Karen was paid $185,662.82. (Later other authorities, including the state board of medical examiners, also checked the work. The state examiners, who were suspicious and extremely thorough, pronounced her work "highly satisfactory.")

Karen had lived up to the contract through a superhuman burst of energy. In rented space in a local hospital, she had scheduled examinations for herself through the evening hours. A platoon of fellow residents moonlighted some evenings and weekends under her direct supervision. At night she herself did the routine laboratory work. She never slept more than three to four hours a night, and some nights she hardly slept at all. She just didn't seem to need sleep, and sometimes she became irritated when she ran out of work to do. A secretary, also moonlighting, came in at 6 A.M. to transcribe Karen's notes and letters from a recording device, and thus the results of the examinations were recorded and referrals made. By 7:30 A.M. on every day scheduled for her, Karen was on duty as a resident. Her supervisors were writing glowing reports about her competence, diligence, and ability to establish rapport with her patients and colleagues. In the end, after all expenses had been paid, the Nerak Clinic showed a profit of $143,741.01.

Karen had never felt happier or more creative, but in fact, her condition was deteriorating. One day, soon after the completion of her contract, her cheerfulness on her hospital ward exceeded the bounds of professional acceptability. Suddenly she burst into song and for half an hour danced up and down the halls. Other staff members tried to calm her, but she lashed out with uncharacteristic irritation. Then she picked up one of the ill children and tried to make him dance with her, telling him that dancing would cure his illness. The senior physician in charge of the ward ordered her to leave the hospital, but because of the fondness and respect everyone felt for Karen, the matter was pursued no further.

That night, unable to sleep and craving excitement, Karen went to a bar. She had several drinks, picked up a man, and took him to her apartment. Thereafter, drinking and having sexual encounters with strangers became a fairly regular activity. One night she entertained three men—sales agents from the same company who were in the city for training. They came back the next two nights. Once she was beaten, and once she was raped.

Looking back on her experience, Karen regarded her promiscuity as the "sickest" of all her behaviors because it was so uncharacteristic of her. But other problems emerged at about the same time. She became highly irritable, snapping out at the slightest provocation. Then irritability merged with euphoria as Karen began a new project, the foundation of a "Universal Healing Institute." The institute was to have a medical school with Karen as dean. Although she was vague when pressed for details, and hard to understand because her rate of speech had increased dramatically, Karen was almost convincing as her ideas tumbled forth. In any case, she could not be pinned down to providing details because she wouldn't tolerate interruptions. She retained an attorney, hired consultants, and leased a block of office space in a prestigious building. She spent hours on the telephone trying to recruit a faculty from medical schools around the world. Several prospective faculty members actually came to visit at Karen's expense. By the time she was forced to accept treatment for her illness, she had spent all of the profits Nerak had earned and was roughly $15,000 in debt.

The end of this phase of Karen's life was brought about by her colleagues and her father. Karen seemed to realize that she should not continue her residency, and she had been appearing at work at irregular hours, often late at night, in order to complete records or do other routine chores. Her supervisor had placed her on sick leave and had assigned her duties to a replacement. Through it all, her colleagues tried to convince her to undergo a comprehensive examination, but Karen insisted she was perfectly well. Eventually, the hospital's senior physician advised her parents to force Karen into treatment.

Her father immediately came to the city. Excited to the point of incoherence, Karen hardly acknowledged her father's presence before resuming an attempt to telephone a prospective faculty member in London. Disheveled, obviously fatigued, and losing weight, Karen seemed to be running on nervous energy alone. Her father tried to convince her to come with him to see a doctor, but he could hardly get her attention, much less hold it. He later paraphrased her responses: "Dad, I love you and of course I'm glad to see you but you can't know. You haven't gone through it with me. Believe me! Where's your shit at anyhow? I've got this vision of the whole goddamn picture, and you are beautiful too but now goddamn it get out of my way. I've got little babies and old people to save. My star is coming from the sky to wipe off all this shit and take me to my place." She had been pacing, talking very rapidly, dismissing with contemptuous gestures her father's attempts to interrupt. But then she lay down on the floor, laughing uproariously. "You didn't squirt me out; I'm queen of the universe and I'm going to fuck God to death."

Sure that his daughter was addicted to drugs, her father agreed to ask a judge to commit her to a hospital for treatment. Karen's father went to the county probate court, where he filled out a form giving his reasons for thinking Karen was mentally ill. Two psychologists appointed by the court examined Karen to determine whether there was "probable cause" to suspect mental illness serious enough to make Karen a danger to herself or others. They quickly agreed that probable cause was present, and the next day a judge ordered Karen brought in for a formal hearing. Two sheriff's deputies took her to a hospital to be held without treatment pending the hearing. Two court-appointed psychiatrists examined her and agreed that she was indeed mentally ill and dangerous to herself— primarily because of poor judgment and inability to adequately attend to her basic hygiene and nutritional needs. Karen's attorney attempted to defeat the petition; a deputy county attorney argued to support it. Karen, agitated, alternated between angry outbursts and coquettish attempts to win the judge over to her side. She was soon removed from the hearing room. The hearing lasted a half-day. Karen was found by the judge to be mentally ill and was committed to a hospital chosen by her father, where she could be held against her will for up to 30 days and treated.

The psychiatrist who treated Karen regarded her as seriously ill. Her hyperactivity was now alternating with periods of near stupor. After the first sleepless night, she refused breakfast and sat immobile in her room. Convinced by Karen's present state and by the history he obtained that Karen's diagnosis was manic-depressive illness and alarmed by her extreme fatigue and poor nutritional state, he recommended immediate treatment with electroconvulsive therapy (ECT). Karen refused to cooperate, and the opinion of a consulting psychiatrist was solicited. She agreed with the treating psychiatrist, and both doctors asked Karen's father to authorize the proposed treatment. He did so, reluctantly.

Over the next 15 days, Karen received eight "shock" treatments, one every other day. After the first treatment, she asked for food and seemed much calmer and more rational for a few hours. Gradually the periods of near normality increased, until, by the seventh treatment, Karen's mood had stabilized and she was fully cooperative. It was agreed that she should be given one more treatment and that thereafter she should take lithium. The court was notified that treatment had been successfully completed, and Karen was discharged from the hospital.

She did not resume her residency. After consulting with her psychiatrist and with the administration of the hospital where she had been a resident, she decided to accept a temporary position in state government inspecting nursing homes. She continued to take lithium.

Karen had two subsequent episodes of illness during the next three years: a major depression much like John's, which was quickly treated with antidepressants, and a period of hyperexcitability and sleeplessness that, though not nearly so prolonged and destructive as her first one, nevertheless disrupted her life. Karen is now happily married and holds a responsible job in medical administration that she finds challenging and fulfilling. For two years her mood has been stable, which, for Karen, means zestful cheerfulness most of the time.

Diagnosis: Bipolar Disorder

Karen's diagnosis, in current terminology, is *bipolar disorder*, one of the major illnesses of mood. An older, more descriptive name is manic-depressive illness. The term *bipolar* describes variation in mood between the two extremes of excessive elation (mania) and depression. Bipolar disorder is less common than major depression. It affects about 0.4 to 0.6 percent of Western populations, males and females equally. Its onset, which may be characterized by either depression or mania, tends to occur in late adolescence; onset after 50 years of age is rare.

Signs and Symptoms

Karen exhibited nearly all the major signs and symptoms of mania. Her mood was euphoric through much of her illness. She was unable to sleep—a nearly universal sign in mania. But unlike John, she didn't try to sleep, because she didn't feel tired. Even after weeks of what would be grossly inadequate sleep for normal people, she did not feel fatigued. Depressed people feel fatigue and complain about lack of sleep. Manic people, if anything, welcome relief from the need to sleep. Like nearly all manics, Karen certainly had increased energy. As is also typical of mania, her judgment was disastrously impaired. In pursuit of a grandiose, impractical scheme, she lost the small fortune she had made doing physical examinations, and she became involved in sexual escapades. These escapades are not unusual in mania; one of the unhappy consequences of a manic episode may be the breakup of a previously stable marriage.

Karen's thought processes were also typical of mania. Her ideas tended to expand without limit as she talked. This tendency, called *flight of ideas*, can be seen in her conversation with her father. Her ideas started on a fairly ordinary level, but they quickly became unreasonable and, finally, outlandish. A key element in mania is grandiosity coupled with wild, bizarre euphoria: Karen's "queen of the universe" statement is an example. A theme can often be discerned in a typical "flight," but the rapid expansion from the commonplace to the exotic or bizarre can be breathtaking.

Another important feature of mania is *pressured speech*—speech so rapid that it seems to race ahead in an effort to keep up with thought. Manics do indeed report "racing," tumbling thoughts that follow one another too quickly to express in speech. Manics are often humorous or entertaining, and people who talk to them may be caught up in the atmosphere they create. This "infectious gaiety" of the manic is unique to mania, so professionals actually use it as a diagnostic hint. When a professional feels empathy with a patient and becomes caught up in euphoric expansiveness, mania suggests itself as a diagnosis.

Though nearly all people with mania sooner or later develop major depression, as Karen did, the reverse is not true. That is, most depressed persons never develop mania. Therefore, there seem to be two principal forms of major mood illnesses: bipolar disorder, which features swings of mood into both depression and mania, and major depression (often called unipolar disorder), in which mania does not occur. In bipolar illness, depression and mania usually occur at different times—hence psychiatrists speak of "episodes"—but in rare cases, the swing is so rapid that the moods virtually merge. Suicidal depression and mania can occur in the same half-hour.

Just how closely linked are bipolar disorder and unipolar depression? They are different forms of illness, yes, but are they different illnesses? The answer to this question is unknown, but some evidence favors a close relationship. For instance, virtually all persons with mania also experience, sooner or later, major depression like John's. There are more subtle hints as well. Bipolar illness typically begins earlier in life than unipolar illness, suggesting that it may be a more severe form of the same illness rather than a separate disorder. (In medicine generally, the earlier the onset of any chronic disease, the greater its severity.) A peculiar feature of mania tends to support this notion. Psychiatrists have observed for decades that often a short depression immediately precedes the onset of mania, which suggests progression from lesser to greater severity. A brief, early depression, you may remember, preceded the period of increasing elation that culminated in Karen's flagrant mania.

It is important to focus on the period of elation experienced before the development of full-blown mania in order to understand the human impact of bipolar illness. Karen's behavior during the time when she was so successfully managing her residency and fulfilling the contract for the medical examinations is technically called *hypomania*, meaning "less than mania." This phase is quite common, and it produces problems unique in medical practice. Far from being dis-ease, such a period of extraordinary energy, optimism, sense of well-being, and productivity is highly valued by those experiencing it. Sometimes, as in Karen's case, astonishing amounts of money are made. Books, plays, and feats of exploration and political success, among many other accomplishments, have been associated with mental states like the one Karen exhibited before her full-blown mania developed.

It is hardly surprising, therefore, that the very last thing some people with bipolar illness want is treatment aimed at terminating their high. Moreover, the optimism and sense of power characteristic of hypomania cause them to minimize the danger of their condition's progressing to full-blown mania, even for those who have experienced it and its disastrous consequences several times. And, in fact, some people with intermittent hypomania never develop mania. This lesser cycling of mood is called *cyclothymia*, and persons affected are called *cyclothymic personalities*. Theirs would appear to be the best of all worlds—except that they are also more likely than normal people to develop major depression.

Prognosis

We have seen that mania reliably portends the development of depression. Her mania having been diagnosed, Karen, her family, and her physicians expected the depression that followed. Beyond that virtually guaranteed development of depression, however, the future course of bipolar illness is less certain. Like major depression, bipolar illness is a cyclic disorder, and a person's cycles often are surprisingly constant. For example, seasonal cycles, with onset in spring and fall, are fairly common.

Mania is a very serious disease if it goes untreated. Extremes of overactivity, energy, and optimism, coupled with impaired judgment, make disaster nearly inevitable. The disaster may be social, in the form of lost friendships, jobs, or marriages; or legal, in the form of criminal charges or lawsuits; or medical, in the form of accidents, illnesses contracted while manic, or complete exhaustion. Before effective treatments were developed, death during manic excitement was not uncommon. Now that treatments are available, the prognosis, when those treatments are applied, is excellent.

Treatment

Bipolar disorder is more difficult to treat than depression, partly because of the psychology of the manic's euphoric high and partly because the disease process, having two phases, is more difficult to manage. Nevertheless, with treatment, most bipolar illness is entirely compatible with both normal life and the creativity that sometimes marks hypomania.

Psychotherapy

Educative psychotherapy is the first line of defense against subsequent episodes of illness. It is the responsibility of professionals to inform those whom they treat and those patient's families about the likelihood of cycles occurring and to teach them how to recognize a cycle early in its course and what to do about it. At first this can be quite unrewarding for all concerned. As a new episode of mania builds, the lessons and promises associated with past episodes are likely to be fast forgotten. But eventually most people with bipolar disorder come to terms with their illness and manage it successfully.

Drug Treatments

Treatments can effectively and promptly terminate bipolar episodes. Electroshock therapy is not often used in mania, but it is effective, as Karen's case demonstrates. However, the use of drugs is far more common. The antidepressant drugs used in major depression (discussed in Chapter 1) are equally effective in treating bipolar depression, and there are two drugs that are especially useful in treating mania.

Lithium

Lithium, a metallic element administered as a salt, is a standard treatment for mania. It is effective during the acute phase of the illness, but achieving an adequate level of the drug in body tissues takes several days. Because mania is a dangerous, even life-threatening disease, other drugs (usually phenothiazines, described in Chapter 3) are often used for initial sedation and then reduced in dose, or stopped altogether, when lithium's effect is established. Lithium also prevents or mitigates future attacks of mania, and it probably does the same for depression.

The precise action of lithium on nerve cells is not known. The use of lithium for mania was discovered accidentally by an Australian doctor who was testing the drug as a treatment for heart disease. But perhaps that should not count as the original discovery: Some of the most famous curative mineral waters the world over contain large amounts of lithium.

As is true of many drugs used in medicine, the concentration of lithium in the body must be controlled within narrow limits: above 0.6 milliequivalents per liter of blood serum to prevent recurrence, above 1.0 milliequivalents per liter to treat acute mania. Toxic signs begin at concentrations of about 1.5 milliequivalents per liter. Because the toxic levels of lithium are close to the therapeutic levels, the concentration of lithium in blood must be checked frequently as the dose increases. The dose needed to achieve therapeutic levels may be as low as 600 milligrams daily or as high as 2400 milligrams (or even more). Happily, once a level is established for a given person, the same dose usually maintains that level, so testing can be minimized.

Everyone who takes lithium should know the signs of toxicity. The first sign is generally upset digestion—nausea, vomiting, diarrhea. A mild tremor of the hands may be bothersome at ordinary doses. At dangerous doses, the tremor usually becomes coarse and exaggerated. Drowsiness, weakness, and lack of coordination are other signs of early toxicity. Staggering gait, blurred vision, and buzzing in the ears signal immediate danger.

Lithium definitely can harm unborn children (it is known to be associated with heart defects) and should not be taken during pregnancy. If a woman discovers that she is pregnant, she should stop taking the drug immediately. Better, if having a baby is even a possibility, lithium should not be used.

Because bipolar illness can be so devastating, lithium treatment, once established, is generally continued indefinitely. There are no recognized long-term detrimental effects, but since the first use of lithium, suspicion has focused on its effect on the kidney and thyroid gland. As a safety measure, many physicians obtain laboratory tests of kidney and thyroid function at intervals during treatment with lithium.

Carbamazepine (Tegretol)

This drug, which has been tested less thoroughly than lithium, is marketed as an anticonvulsant, but it also appears to be effective as an antimanic agent. As with lithium, the dose must be individualized, 800 to 1500 milligrams a day is usually needed. Side effects, especially dizziness and drowsiness, are often present, but they are mild, fleeting, and not often troublesome. The most effective use of this drug has not yet been determined, but it may become a standard supplement to lithium whenever lithium alone is less than optimally effective. There is no information about risk to unborn children. Over the past few years, other preparations in the same class as carbamazepine have become available, making this an active and promising area of pharmacologic research.

There are a few cases that simply do not respond to available treatments. Some bipolar patients develop a chronic mood disorder that treatment only partially relieves. Sometimes the cycling is so rapid that treatments cannot keep up. Some affected persons present a constellation of signs and symptoms that at times fulfills all diagnostic criteria for depression or mania and at other times suggests schizophrenia. This condition warrants a separate diagnosis, *schizoaffective disorder*. This diagnosis is confusing and controversial, because it is not clear exactly how schizoaffective disorder is related to either schizophrenia or mood disorder. It also can be most difficult to treat. Current practice is to treat for both mood disorder and schizophrenia according to the signs and symptoms present at a given time. This is possible in many instances, but it is hard to manage. Overall, however, well over 90 percent of cases of bipolar disorder respond very well to treatment, once the affected person agrees that treatment is needed and consistently cooperates with it.

■ *If You Think You Have Bipolar Disorder*

The main thing is not to be swept along by mood changes in either direction. This isn't easy. While we all seem to be wired so that it takes intense effort to prevent emotions from overriding rational thought, you are especially vulnerable to this when your mood is either high or low. Your main defense is to learn what changes signal the onset of mood swings in your particular case. The first step is to learn what changes signal the onset of mood swings in your case. The earlier in the process the signals occur, the better. By the time manic euphoria or deep depression develops, it may be too late to prevent damage. Often, disturbed sleep is a reliable clue. Some people who are taking lithium say that they can spot an incipient swing into mania because they feel as though a lid—the lithium—were holding them down. Use such clues to tell you that it is time for an extra visit to the doctor—and for added control from you. Get help with that added control if you can. Find another person (your spouse perhaps, or a sibling or a friend) to whom, when an agreed-upon sign of illness appears, you will yield control. This is hard to do. None of us can find more than a few people during life whom we can trust to that extent, but on the other hand, we all have to trust another person occasionally. As a person with bipolar illness, recognize that you have a special need to trust. Resolve to place it wisely, honor it, and keep reminding yourself of it.

■ *If Someone Close to You Has Bipolar Disorder*

You have a close relationship with a person who is likely to be creative, energetic, and charming when well, and nearly unbearable when ill. To cope, you too must learn to recognize the signs of impending mood swings. One sign that affected persons themselves are not usually aware of is the rate of their speech, which tends to speed up in mania and to slow down with depression. This is a reliable sign in many affected persons. Your aim is to use the clues you discover to avoid extreme swings in mood and to prevent swings that do occur from doing damage.

Rely on professional help to soften the swings. Increasing drug dosage for a few days, or even just scheduling a few extra counseling visits, will often accomplish this. To minimize damage, first recognize that behaviors such as manic irritability, arrogance, and maddening energy, as well as depressive isolation and whining self-depreciation, are temporary manifestations of illness, as impersonal as fever or sniffles. Then try to obtain agreement that when an early sign of mood shift occurs, such as a change in sleep pattern or rate of speech, you will take over making decisions and will organize daily schedules, including appointments with health care professionals. This may not work at first; experience with the effects of the disease may be needed. But eventually, most people affected with bipolar disorder do agree to accept help. Keep trying. Never abuse whatever trust you are given. Keep yourself under control. In particular, avoid being caught up in the manic's infectious gaiety. If you go along a little way, you will find it hard to stop. Be firm and matter-of-fact as you apply the brakes. Most of all, keep in mind that the episode will pass and full recovery will ensue.

▪ Judicial Commitment ▪

The process of judicial commitment is one of the most controversial in modern psychiatric practice because it limits personal liberty and often imposes treatment against the will of one held to be mentally ill. The process is governed by state laws, which vary, and its application is modified by local custom, the professional personnel available to the court responsible, and the size of the community.

The law has long recognized the right of individuals to accept or refuse medical or surgical treatment, even when their lives are at risk. An exception occurs when the brain is the organ impaired. The brain is needed for rational decision making. If one's brain is not functioning normally, can one make decisions in one's own best interest? To this question, the law's answer has been no, and legislatures have written statutes giving judges authority to commit persons found to be mentally ill to hospitals where they may be held against their will and, in some cases, forcibly treated. In short, the court is empowered to substitute its judgment for judgment impaired by brain disease.

Until major changes in the laws governing commitment were made during the 1960s and early 1970s, the process was quite simple. A petition was submitted to a court, usually the county probate court. In theory, anyone could do this, but usually a relative initiated the process. If a relative was not available, someone else likely to come into contact with ill persons—such as a doctor, lawyer, or police officer—filed the petition. If the judge found some basis for believing that significant illness was present, physicians (psychiatrists, if available) were asked to give opinions. The judge then found that mental illness either was present or was not present. If illness was determined to be present, the judge committed the person to medical custody, usually in a hospital. The process was informal and swift.

Impelled by the civil rights activism of the 1960s, the commitment process became a focus of controversy. There had been a rash of newspaper and television exposés about persons committed to state institutions after perfunctory court procedures and kept there against their will for years. In response, legislatures enacted laws greatly changing the process of judicial commitment. Now, after a petition is filed, a screening team employed by the court visits the "prospective patient," as the object of the petition has become known, in order to determine whether there is "probable cause"— meaning reason to believe that major mental illness is present and that voluntary treatment is not a practical option. If probable cause is found, a formal trial is held. The prospective patient, who is present, is represented by an attorney. Witnesses are sworn, examined, and cross-examined. At this stage it is not enough simply to find illness present. Prospective patients must also be found to be an immediate danger to themselves or others because they have engaged in some overt, physically threatening act or, in some states, because they are unable to obtain food or shelter, or both. Commitment, if ordered, must be made to a facility providing the "least restrictive environment" appropriate to the patient's condition. The process has become extremely complex, adversarial, time-consuming, and expensive. In an effort to mold reality into armchair visions of a perfect world, the legal niceties surrounding due process are scrupulously enforced, thus theoretically eliminating any possibility of human error. The result has been to turn the process into a criminal trial with ill persons as defendants and their relatives as accusers, rather than a forum in which, ideally, all parties seek to secure the most humane and effective treatment for an ill person.

I have practiced medicine in four states, before and after the reforms of the 1960s, and have assisted in the commitment process hundreds of times. Although I do not believe many people were once railroaded into hospitals, I think the process *did* need repair. The fairness of the time-honored process depended on the competence and goodwill of those involved. The humaneness and wisdom of the judges were the main safeguards. Of course, not all judges are humane and competent, and some are neither. Moreover, the judge's responsibility boiled down to informally enforcing community standards of behavior. This was not unreasonable when communities tended to be small, homogeneous, and stable. But community standards cannot even be defined, let alone informally enforced, in today's American society. In addition, the older standards were sometimes intolerant of the merely eccentric and of harmless public nuisances. Forced hospitalization is a major infringement of liberty that must be treated with utmost seriousness. Safeguards are needed.

However, as seems to be inevitable in reforms of human institutions, the pendulum has swung too far. Scrupulous enforcement of the minutiae of due process and a relative disregard for human problems have occasioned the unwise and unfeeling release of far too many "prospective patients" who go on to commit suicide or to wander the streets insane. Recently, common sense seems to have begun modifying what the courts actually do. Possibly a new equilibrium is evolving that will serve the real best interests of ill persons and their families. But this essential change is proceeding fitfully and is far from complete.

■■■

■ *If You Are Considering Judicial Commitment of a Relative*

Yours is a heartbreaking responsibility. If you are the nearest relative, no one else can successfully initiate commitment unless you fully agree and cooperate; even if you do not take the first steps, the major responsibility to consent will eventually be yours. So there is no escape. If you believe your relative is ill and a danger to herself or himself or to others, you will have to go to the probate court of your county and give reasons supporting your belief.

Do not be afraid to approach the court, even if you are not sure what to do. The people you will see when you first go to the probate court are most understanding and helpful. Go talk to them. They will respect your confidence, so you have nothing to lose. You will receive sound advice and, if you decide to go ahead with a petition, expert help in filing it. But from that time onward, you will find that the civil rights of the prospective patient—your relative—have by far the highest priority.

You will be asked to obtain a supporting statement from a physician if one has seen your relative recently. If not, you will be asked to make every reasonable effort to get a physician involved. Court-appointed examiners will then consider all available evidence, including an interview with your relative to determine whether probable cause exists. These examiners, the prepetition team, will submit a recommendation to the judge. Although appeal of their recommendation is theoretically possible, it is not practical in most jurisdictions. If the examiners do not find probable cause, your petition will be dismissed. If probable cause is found, you will have to appear in court and may be called as a witness to testify in the presence of your relative. He or she will have an attorney who will try to defeat the petition. Expect to be cross-examined. Plan on spending a full day in court; any appeals will demand additional time. Even if commitment is ordered, refusal of treatment may become an issue. In many states, authorization of treatment against a patient's will now requires further appearances in court.

The question I am most often asked is "If I go to court, will my loved one always hold it against me? I'm afraid he will hate me forever." I have seen this outcome, but it is rare. Most often your relative emerges from treatment grateful to you or at least understands why you felt forced to take action. More important, you will both almost surely lose if you delay. Most mental illness does not go away by itself. Delay will mean exposure to risks— not only risks of physical injury, but also risks at work and risks of disruptive behavior that must later be lived down. Reputations can be destroyed. Most of all, ill persons are usually frightened and miserable. It is cruel to look the other way. There are risks no matter what you do, but taking action is most often far less risky than doing nothing.

Part

2

THINKING

■■■

To the founders of psychiatry, some diseases seemed set apart because they caused progressive, permanent loss of higher mental functions. In these diseases, the mind "de-mented," so they became known as dementing illnesses. They fall into two major categories, which are the topics of the next two chapters.

One of these categories, which is addressed in Chapter 4, contains Alzheimer's disease and several other diseases that produce nearly the same effects. Progressive losses of memory, of ability to reason abstractly, and of judgment characterize these diseases. There is also loss of brain tissue.

The other category includes schizophrenia, which is probably not one disease but several that we cannot now separate. Memory remains intact in schizophrenia, and ability to reason abstractly is not so obviously impaired. Nevertheless, to early psychiatrists it seemed evident that schizophrenia was a progressive dementia, though a dementia mainly of affect rather than of intellectual attributes. Hence their descriptive term *affective dementia.* These early psychiatrists observed that unlike John and Karen, whose affective capacities returned to what they were before they became ill, many (probably most) people afflicted with schizophrenia did not return completely to their baseline condition after an attack of illness. Modern investigations have shown this picture to be oversimplified in that slight progressive loss of function may occur in some affective illnesses. But the broad generalization is valid for practical purposes: Schizophrenia implies progressive marring of personality.

This section begins with schizophrenia because it is the prototypic mental illness. When the general public imagines "craziness," or Hollywood tries to depict it, or politicians deplore the large numbers of hospital beds still occupied by the mentally ill, they are thinking primarily of schizophrenia. Because the disease progresses over much of a lifetime, an instructive case history must cover decades instead of the few years that were sufficient for John and Karen.

3

Schizophrenia

❏ *George*

George had become unusually quiet and retiring for a 17-year-old. He had been known as a mildly unsettled boy, moody and sometimes oversensitive, but most often he seemed to be normally active and was accepted by his friends. His mischievous streak was well known to his teachers. He was a steady performer on his high school basketball team and a second clarinet in the band.

At first, the changes in George's behavior were hard for others to identify. For George himself, the most notable feature was that no matter where he was or what he was doing, he felt a strange, gnawing fear. School became particularly painful. In the confusion of the halls and cafeteria, the playful, vigorous moves of his young peers sometimes seemed for a moment to be purposeful physical threats. Half-heard sounds seemed to mock or threaten him. George knew that these things were not really true, but he was still afraid. By moving quietly along the school's corridors and trying not to attract attention, he was able to keep his distress at barely tolerable levels. But this relief had a price. Gradually, he interacted less and less with his classmates and teachers, until his presence went largely unnoticed. His academic work deteriorated. His B average slipped until he was getting C's and D's.

George's parents had divorced when he was 4 years old; a few years later his father died of multiple sclerosis. His mother, with whom he lived, had worked for several years in the county sheriff's tax office, where she enjoyed security and a comfortable salary. Her life centered on her church, where she spent much of her free time. Always devout, since her divorce she had developed increasingly intense religious feelings that had led her to join a small evangelical sect. She recognized that life was not going well for George; perhaps God was testing him. But she paid little attention to his developing problem.

After two difficult months, George's fear slowly lessened and his sense of well-being returned to near its usual level. He continued in the school band but withdrew gratefully from basketball because of a serious toenail infection. That gave him time to try out for a part in the senior class play. Acting somehow came easy to George. He won a major role in which he was an outstanding success. By the time the play closed, George had earned a new popularity with his peers, and his confidence was almost completely restored.

Just before graduation from high school, George experienced an intense fright. While sitting alone at home at the kitchen table, he noticed that a unit on the electric stove had been left on and was glowing red. To him, the glow suddenly became terrifying. It first seemed to shoot sparks at him. Then it moved toward him, taking a human form—"the Devil alive!" George recoiled, horrified. He sat transfixed for several seconds before he could bolt into the living room. He was sure that some trick was being played on his brain. He remembered smelling something that he had taken for a food odor, but it suddenly occurred to him that there must have been poison gas in the house. That thought immediately became a conviction. He *knew* poison gas had been present; no other explanation was possible. Afraid to return to the kitchen, he left the burner on and shied away from the stove for weeks. He had read that miners used canaries to detect poison gas. He thought about getting one but decided that would be cruel. It was a warm spring, so he kept opening windows, which his mother kept closing. She didn't ask why he was doing this and he didn't explain.

A few days later he saw a sign in the window of a bakery: *Stale Sale*. Immediately, George knew that the sign was a message. "Stale" publicly proclaimed him to be a homosexual, and "sale" meant he was seeking to buy sex. He had had no sexual experience, and what urges he had known had been heterosexual. But he knew with absolute conviction what the sign "really" meant.

More such signals appeared to George. A television news reporter sent coded messages. Often these were jokes that caused George to laugh to himself. His mother would sometimes ask him what was so funny, but he shrugged off her questions with a look that suggested she was only pretending not to understand. Of course she really didn't understand, but she did not inquire further. Instead she increasingly ignored her son. He never asked himself who or what might be sending him messages, but he felt the return of the fear.

After he graduated from high school, George enlisted in the Navy. It was not that he wanted to, but he just saw no other option and had the idea that he wanted to study radar. The television news reporter sent him messages signifying that he approved of George's enlistment. Once George reached a Navy training center, however, his fear—intensified by novelty and confusion—again became terror. One afternoon, he suddenly "knew" that one of the cooks was Satan and that his training group's flag was that of the devil's. That evening at dinner, George was sure at least one of the items on his tray had been poisoned. But he was also sure that refusing to eat would attract attention and give him away. He ate only potatoes.

After dinner, male and female voices began to speak to him. Twice by reflex he exclaimed, "Listen!" The first time, the recruit in the bed next to him responded, "Listen to what?" The second time he just looked strangely at George. One of the voices told George, "That guy can't hear me," but George somehow knew that without being told. He didn't know where the voices were coming from, but he knew that some external power—perhaps Satan, perhaps someone or something else—was responsible. Most of the time, the voices commented on the barracks life around him and often on his fellow trainees. One voice would say, "That guy is ugly." "Yeah, an ugly dog, a real hound dog," said another. Sometimes they instructed him, "Go hit that one." "No, just watch him; he's only a queer queer," said another voice, which made George giggle. The voices giggled too.

George hardly slept that night because he had to keep watch on a fire extinguisher that a voice told him was Satan's hiding place. By the next morning, he did not make sense when he talked. He babbled, "Got one to seven—see, the life in the drain—it's all butaco." At other times he looked up attentively as if listening to his voices; sometimes he giggled. During morning cleanup, he thought he saw his "life stuff dragged by Satan into the mop bucket." He ran screaming down the street in front of the barracks.

Surprisingly, George's bizarre behavior attracted little attention for several days. He managed to go through the motions of a demanding training program, even though the voices increasingly occupied his attention. His fellow trainees could not help noticing how George was acting, but they tried hard to ignore it because they sensed that George was not to be understood. Unapproachable, afraid, and preoccupied with the products of his distorted brain, George was allowed to melt into the background.

Of course this couldn't last. One day, when confronted by an officer after wandering away from a marching formation, George smiled vacantly as he spoke about how he was resisting Satan's lusts. He was taken to the base hospital, where a diagnosis of schizophrenia was made. He was given Stelazine (a major tranquilizing drug), which lessened his fear and, after a few days, seemed to make the voices go away. More precisely, George now realized that the voices were actually his own thoughts. He felt sluggish, but he was no longer so obviously disturbed, and within a week of his admission to the base hospital, George, with an extra dose of Stelazine for the trip, was on his way to a hospital near his home. His medical discharge was being processed.

For the last few hours of his trip, George noticed that his neck seemed to be twisting to his right and up and that his eyes moved in the same direction. With effort, he could bring his head and eyes to their usual position, but when he relaxed his concentration they would not stay there. By the time he arrived at the hospital, his muscles had become so sore that he felt his head and eyes were locked in their rightward and upward deviations. George did not suspect that his new problem was a side effect of Stelazine.

At the hospital George finally had a little good luck. The admitting doctor recognized the cause of his neck and eye deviation. An antidote, the antihistamine drug Benadryl given by injection into a vein, immediately relieved him, although the muscles remained tender for several hours.

A new doctor took over his case. He reviewed the history sent with George and did his own examination. He agreed with the diagnosis of schizophrenia but changed the drug treatment from Stelazine to Trilafon, a drug in the same class with which the doctor was more familiar. George was also given Akineton, a drug used to counter the side effects. There were other treatments. He saw the doctor three times a week for psychotherapy. Every day there were meetings—treatment groups, occupational therapy, "community meetings" attended by all patients and staff. Everyone tried very hard to understand George and to help him to understand himself.

George tried, too. He attended every meeting but found real participation impossible. Although he was no longer hearing voices and could think clearly, he still felt lethargic, as if drugged (which, of course, he was). He was also uncomfortably stiff, especially when he tried to move quickly. At the same time, he sometimes experienced such painful restlessness that he felt driven to pace up and down the halls and around the dayroom.

In the group meetings George was continually asked what he was feeling: "How did that make you feel?" "What did you feel then?" In fact, he felt nothing most of the time. However, the hospital staff thought he was getting better, mainly because he no longer acted as though he were hearing voices or thinking crazy thoughts. He was eating well, gaining weight, and looking healthier. He himself was grateful for the disappearance of the voices and especially for the lessening of the terror he had lived with so long. But he also felt "dead" or "drugged," as he described his feelingless state. One day he found a pin and began running it through his skin again and again—through a finger, through a fold of skin picked up on his forearm, then through his cheek. Actually, George just wanted to feel something, but he couldn't organize his thoughts well enough to explain this to the horrified nurse who discovered him or to his therapy groups, who spent the next two sessions theorizing about his self-mutilation.

Twice each day, a nurse brought George's medicine served in a little paper cup. In a new effort to make something happen, he began to mouth his pills and later spit them out. By the next day he began to feel more alive. His joints moved better, he was more alert, and his evening meal tasted good. The next morning he awakened feeling zestful and looking forward to the day. However, two days later his problems began to return—first messages from the television, then a firm conviction that a nurse was Satan's mistress and that the pair were having intercourse right in front of him, though he could never catch them at it. The next evening the voices resumed.

The staff saw that George was getting worse and immediately suspected the reason. They began administering his medicine in liquid form, and they watched him swallow. He quickly lapsed into his state of lethargy and physical discomfort, but regained a relatively clear brain. In a group meeting a student nurse asked him how, during the time when he was not taking his medicine, he could possibly have believed that Satan had again appeared. She reasoned that because George had told the group about Satan's previous appearances and realized that these were "sick" ideas, he should have realized that Satan's reappearance was also an illusion. "Good point," he thought, but he had no answer. He had "known" that Satan was in the fire extinguisher. Later he knew that this belief was erroneous, but when Satan returned, George again "knew" that the devil's presence was horribly real. The staff proceeded to direct the group toward discussion of medicines and the importance of taking them. George almost agreed, but not quite. Whether to be sick or to be drugged made a hard choice.

All through his stay in the hospital, people had talked to him about work. George, in one of the spunky moments that seemed to be more frequent, named this effort "get the slob a job." He took tests, filled out applications, and was interviewed. Work was a theme in therapy sessions with his groups, with his doctor, and with a vocational counselor. He was enrolled in an eight-week program that would train him to become a small-appliance repairman.

Job planning was just one of the preparations designed to make it possible for George to leave the hospital. George had been there nearly two months—long enough, everyone agreed. He was better. He no longer heard voices, and best by far, his fear had lessened dramatically. He still felt lethargic, but much less so. His mother had been visiting almost every week and had become involved in "family therapy." In family therapy sessions, George, his mother, and one or two staff members (usually a social worker and a nurse) discussed problems that had come up or were likely to come up between George and his mother. Neither he nor his mother said much. He felt nothing was important enough to raise as an issue, and except when religious themes were mentioned, his mother was ill at ease among all the professionals. The conscientious staff worked hard trying to define problems and solutions. Sometimes they thought they had made some progress, but in truth, no one—not the doctor nor the staff nor George nor his mother—had any idea what would really be helpful.

When George at last was discharged from the hospital, his treatment was to continue at a community mental health clinic. But when he went to the center, he discovered it hardly existed except on paper. A secretary and a social worker were working full time, but no psychiatrist was available. A family doctor came to the clinic one afternoon a week to write prescriptions.

Even so, George's vocational training was paying off. He still felt "blah," as he often said, but he was learning to fix things and found tinkering a relatively pleasant way to spend his days. His work was slow, and sometimes he made mistakes so careless that they were hard to understand. But he was improving, and by the time he graduated, had become reasonably competent. The school helped him land a job as a helper in a large warehouse managed by an electrical contractor who made and repaired neon signs. He began as a marginal worker, but before long he had demonstrated enough initiative and competence to be trusted with sizable installations. In fact, he was feeling much better. He even contacted a couple of high school classmates and joined the company of an amateur theater. Again he landed an important part in a play and, for the first time in months, began to enjoy himself.

George remained well for nearly a year. He took small doses of Trilafon, worked, and stayed with his mother. His social life centered on the theater, where he had won other major roles. The balance of his free time was spent watching television. Then, for no apparent reason, illness returned. First came a few days of increasing fear, then "signs," dozens of them, from television, from almost anywhere. For example, a co-worker came to work with a new red plastic lunchbox. Suddenly George "knew" that Satan had caused the co-worker to buy the lunchbox as a sign to the world that he (George) was homosexual. A day later the voices began again. The doctor increased George's medicine, but he only got worse. He re-entered the hospital, where he stayed for almost 12 weeks.

Over the next 15 years, George was in and out of hospitals and worked only sporadically. Sometimes he was terribly ill, hallucinating almost constantly, but more often he was relatively well. He would take medicine when very distressed, then stop when he felt drugged. About midway through this period, his mother had a stroke and died after spending two months in a nursing home. George began to live in a succession of halfway houses, which provided room and board and various degrees of supervision for mental patients. These homes had sprung up in the vacuum left by state hospitals which had been closing or greatly reducing their populations.

At rare intervals, George became visibly angry. For no under-standable reason, he would abruptly begin lecturing a character in a television serial, or, apparently incensed by an item in a newscast, he would pace about, loudly arguing with no one. Occasionally he lashed out at others around him. But always he would abruptly stop raging and again present a wooden expression that seldom changed. When George seemed to be getting much worse, the staff of the halfway house would take him to the emergency room of the county hospital or to a state hospital. Twice he was committed to the state hospital that served his geographic area. There too, the staff tried hard to find better answers for George's problems. None was found. George was given medication and discharged within a few days. The hospital was grossly understaffed and simply had to make room for newly committed patients.

A major problem for all of those who tried to help George was his apparent lack of motivation. There seemed to be nothing that he wanted except food and coffee. Neither earning money in a sheltered workshop nor working for chips exchangeable for television time and sweets changed his performance. He didn't refuse to work or argue about assignments. He might even begin a job, but then he would apparently lose interest and just sit. Sometimes volunteers or (during early years) people who had known George from his days in the electric sign shop would take him on excursions. He always went, but he seemed to be just going through the motions. He said thank you, as he knew he should, but he felt nothing—no twinge of gratitude, no resentment, nothing at all. When visitors stopped coming, no one heard him complain.

Several times George left halfway houses and managed to travel long distances. He apparently spent most of his time as a homeless person, living outdoors. By this time he was receiving disability payments from Social Security, but most of the money went to cover his cost of room and board; he certainly had nothing extra for travel. Usually he would turn up at a public assistance office, where he was given clean clothing, a little money, and a bus ticket home.

After returning from one such trip, George was found wandering in a suburban shopping mall, unkempt and talking wildly to himself. A new commitment proceeding was begun, but by this time the criteria had been changed, and involuntary commitment required unequivocal evidence of his being a danger to himself or others. It was ruled that George, though a public nuisance, was not dangerous within the meaning of the law. He was released. A week later his body was found beneath a bridge. He had been murdered with a heavy stone found nearby, apparently for the $20 he had obtained that day from a public assistance office.

Diagnosis: Schizophrenia

George had schizophrenia. His illness was more rapidly progressive and less responsive to treatment than average, but then every expert would advance a different definition of the course of average or typical schizophrenia. The signs, symptoms, and disabilities produced by schizophrenia vary more widely than those of any other mental illness.

Schizophrenia affects about eight out of every thousand persons who live to their early forties. All the world's populations, be they industrial, hunter-gatherer, urban, or rural, exhibit about the same rate of this illness. On average, males fall ill earlier in life, but females catch up later; by midlife, equal proportions are affected. The average age at onset is about 27, but the illness may begin in adolescence or in adult life until about age 50. Onset after that is rare. Most authorities think that schizophrenia is more than one illness and encompasses a whole group of diseases. Just as "fever" and "anemia" were once regarded as distinct diseases but were eventually subdivided, so subdivision of schizophrenia will almost certainly come about, although today there is not enough evidence to support any particular reclassification.

George had a fairly typical onset: delusions, hallucinations, and disturbed thinking with consequent bizarre behavior. What happens after onset is quite variable. Most often, as with George, there are remissions—periods during which the disease is quiescent. Thus the disease proceeds in episodes: acute attack followed by recovery, then another acute attack, and so on. Sometimes recovery seems permanent or nearly so; there are no further acute attacks, or widely spaced recurrences are separated by an apparently complete return to normal. But most often recovery is incomplete and each acute attack is followed by increasing disability. This result, known as *chronic schizophrenia,* is the course George's illness took. Finally, there is sometimes just one attack from which there is no recovery. Because onset is early in life and because life expectancy is only slightly reduced, decades of social cripplement commonly result from schizophrenia. The combination of schizophrenia's high incidence and the lengthy disability it inflicts make it one of the world's major public health problems. However, as we will see, new treatments promise to make a real difference in outcome.

Signs and Symptoms

Acute schizophrenia is marked mainly by disturbances in *thinking and perception*. Chronic schizophrenia adds to these disturbances a profound deficit in *affect*. Thinking is divided into two components, content and progression. Because we cannot know directly what another person is thinking, what professionals really mean by "thinking" is what is said in speech.

Thought Content

This component consists of what is thought about. In schizophrenia, abnormal thought content is marked by delusions. Delusions are false beliefs that cannot be corrected in spite of evidence. George's conviction that Satan was in the fire extinguisher is an example. Delusions are not limited to schizophrenia but rather occur in many brain diseases. However, in schizophrenia they are so common that they are nearly essential to the diagnosis.

Schizophrenics describe delusions as forming instantly; a conjecture comes to mind and is immediately "known" to be true beyond any doubt. That delusions cannot be corrected has been discovered by many well-meaning friends and beginning mental health professionals who have tried their best to disprove a delusional belief. When I was a psychiatric resident, one of my first patients believed that the menu posted on a bulletin board in the hospital cafeteria contained that day's messages from the board of directors of the company he worked for. I knew that the menu was published a week in advance, and I obtained a copy; it was dated the week before but contained that day's menu. When I confronted my patient with this proof that the menu could not have contained daily messages for him, he was not even surprised, let alone convinced of the error of his belief. "Well, that means they predicted today's events pretty well," he said. "But if they had needed to send a different message, they would have."

Delusions take innumerable forms. An affected person may be absolutely convinced that his or her thoughts are being read by aliens and broadcast on television or that he or she is a victim of witchcraft, is a target of organized crime, is being spied on by neighbors, has a brain made of nickel, or is the target of laser beams that stimulate genitalia. Any aspect of the environment may provoke a delusional belief. A gesture may be interpreted as a sign; a cough or crossed legs may signal to others that the affected person is perverted or dishonest. When present, delusions can dominate conscious life, excluding other thoughts. Delusions tend to be multiple, one following immediately upon another, but there is often a central core delusion around which all of the others revolve. "The pope is trying to silence me. That woman over there is his agent—see the way she has her hand in her lap? That means that if I tell what I know, they are going to get me for masturbation."

Delusions were once seen as a window on mental life. It seemed obvious to early psychiatrists that there must be some psychic logic underlying delusions. For example, a man's belief that covert massages in television broadcasts accuse him of sexual exploitation of children was thought likely to be based on his "unconscious" wishes. Such speculations have proved misleading. No one knows why delusions occur or what shapes their content.

Progression of Thought

Schizophrenic thinking processes are more difficult to define than thought content. Professionals do agree that something is wrong with the way the brains of some schizophrenics process thoughts. This defect is easy to characterize when thinking is grossly fragmented or irrelevant to the situation, as it was at times in George's illness. Though easily recognizable, milder forms of disordered progression of thought (such as "wooly vagueness," a term found in clinical literature) are difficult to describe and thus hard to formulate as diagnostic signs. Today's professionals do not emphasize progression of thought in diagnosing schizophrenia. This major change has occurred over the past decade. Learning to recognize "loosening of associations" (to the satisfaction of one's supervisor) was once a rite of passage for psychiatrists in training. Today, flagrant disordered progression of thought is noted and given due consideration, but it does not occupy center stage.

Perceptions

Hallucinations are common in schizophrenia. An hallucination is a sensory perception that does not correspond to external stimuli. Any sensory system can be involved: Hallucinations can be visual, tactile (touch), olfactory (smell), gustatory (taste), or auditory (hearing). Any type of hallucination may occur in schizophrenia, but auditory hallucinations are by far the most common. These can be of any sound—music, moans of torture victims seeming to come from mirrors, gunshots—but in schizophrenia, the sounds are most often the voices of one or more persons, usually identifiable as male or female, often associated with names. Sometimes, but not usually, the voices are those of people the ill person knows. Most often they keep up a running commentary on events and people in the environment, but sometimes they give commands: "Stay away!" "Forget that!" Hallucinatory voices marking severe schizophrenia often refer to the affected person in the third person, either by name or as "him" or "her."

To one listening to a schizophrenic describe auditory hallucinations, it often seems obvious that the voices must be the thoughts of the person experiencing them. What the voices say seems understandable when interpreted in that way. But to the ill person, the voices nearly always seem to come from outside the brain—from the air through radio waves, from the walls through hidden loudspeakers, from a radio receiver maliciously installed in a filled tooth. Sometimes the process is reversed: The affected person perceives that the voices express his or her own thoughts and is sure some external force is broadcasting them aloud for the whole world to hear.

It is always astonishing when very intelligent schizophrenics admit that they cannot suggest an external physical basis for their hallucinations but nevertheless absolutely insist that there is one. A parallel phenomenon is equally astonishing. Sometimes, as in George's case, a person recovering from an acute episode recognizes that hallucinatory voices originate internally. Then, if over the next few hours a mild setback in recovery occurs, that same individual may again blame external forces.

Chronic Schizophrenia

Between acute attacks of schizophrenia, a gradual worsening often becomes apparent. This process does not prominently involve greater intensity of delusions or hallucinations. Rather, it leads to a defect in affect, those moment-to-moment changes in internal emotion described in Part 1. The result is called the chronic *deficit state* or *residual state*. The changes of chronic schizophrenia develop slowly. It is hard to follow their progress with any precision, but over time, the insidious destruction of personality becomes obvious.

First comes a *blunting of affect*. Schizophrenics seem to progressively lose their ability to experience subtler shades of feeling: empathy for the situation of another, finer gradations of humor, friendly regard for others, the warmth of closeness, the exhilaration of competition. Most disabling is the slow development of an apparent lack of capacity to feel pleasure, a condition called *anhedonia*. The disease seems to cripple the reward systems of the brain so that a chronic schizophrenic does not feel pleasure but rather is indifferent to the sweetness of life. Compliments from another and the rewards of work, for instance, evoke decreasing emotional responses—and eventually none at all. A person with schizophrenia told me, "I used to love autumn winds with blowing leaves and so I went out and walked by the river. I built up thoughts and imagined scenes just as if I were feeling again. But then I realized that I was only forcing myself to pretend that my insides were intense and feeling. I felt the wind on my skin, but inside, nothing happened to me."

It is this poverty of feeling that apparently accounts for the lack of motivation observed in chronic schizophrenia. Efforts at rehabilitation fail because a crippled internal-reward system no longer provides any reason to expend effort.

As the finer shades of emotional life are lost, exaggeration of more primitive emotions occurs. Anger and fear, especially fear, are expressed with excessive intensity. Coarse outbursts occur without apparent cause and are rarely followed by any actions implied by the emotion. George exhibited this during his stays in halfway houses. And as one gets to know schizophrenics, one comes to realize that a main experience of their lives is fear—unreasoning, constant fear.

The final stage is reached when the only emotions expressed are rare outbursts of fear or anger. By then, affect is graphically described as "wooden." Through it all, intelligence, in the sense of cognitive ability and memory, remains intact. Schizophrenics know what is happening.

Prognosis

The prognosis in schizophrenia is highly variable. A fairly accurate rule of thumb says that one-third of cases have a good outcome, one-third a poor outcome, and one-third an outcome that falls somewhere in between. A good outcome consists of one or two acute attacks with undetectable or barely detectable chronic changes. A poor outcome is characterized by nearly constant hospitalization. (We would locate George toward the more severe end of the middle group.) The number and intensity of acute attacks with delusions, hallucinations, and disorganized thinking are not nearly so important predictors of outcome as whether the disease becomes chronic. Acute schizophrenia responds well to available treatments, but there is no satisfactory treatment for chronicity. Decades of study have yielded some predictors of outcome. On the average, good outcome is associated with

1. Acute onset as opposed to gradual, insidious onset. (George's onset was of the latter kind.)

2. A clear precipitating event. This can be a major personal loss—a death, for example. But a job promotion with added responsibility is another frequent precipitant.

3. Mood disturbance, usually a depression, associated with the acute attack.

4. High intelligence. In general in psychiatric illness, the higher the IQ, the better the prognosis. This is particularly true in schizophrenia.

5. Good premorbid adjustment. The further a person has progressed in school, and the more developed a person's social and vocational skills before the onset of illness, the better the outcome.

Treatment

Today the treatment of schizophrenia is based on five main classes of drugs known as *major tranquilizers*, or *neuroleptics*. They are listed in

SOME DRUGS THAT ARE EFFECTIVE IN TREATING SCHIZOPHRENIA

Class	Trade Name	Chemical Name	Typical Daily Dose (milligrams)
Phenothiazines			
	Prolixin[1,2]	Fluphenazine	10
	Stelazine[1]	Trifluoperazine	30
	Trilifon[1]	Perphenazine	40
	Mellaril	Thioridazine	400
	Thorazine[1]	Chlorpromazine	500
Butyrophenones			
	Haldol[1,2]	Haloperidol	20
Thioxanthenes			
	Navane[1]	Thiothixene	20
	Taractan[1]	Chlorprothixene	150
Dibenzoxazepines			
	Loxitane	Loxapine	100
	Clozaril	Clozapine	350
Dihydroindolones			
	Moban	Molindone	75

[1] Also available in injectable form.
[2] Also available in long-lasting (10 to 14 days) injectable form.

the table above. With respect to their effect on the major signs and symptoms of schizophrenia, there is disappointingly little difference among them, but there are wide differences in dosage, relative sedating properties, and the frequency of various side effects.

The basic action of all these drugs is the same: They block transmission of nerve impulses via the neurotransmitter dopamine by occupying dopamine receptors on postsynaptic membranes. (See the figure on page 27.) There is no doubt that these drugs are effective against the main features of acute schizophrenia. They suppress the delusions, hallucinations, and flagrantly disorganized thinking. More than any other factor or combination of factors, these drugs have made life outside a hospital possible for thousands of people.

What else these drugs do is not so clear and not so obviously beneficial. Authorities now agree that they do not improve an established chronic residual state; neither motivation nor anhedonia (lack of capacity to experience pleasure) is changed. Whether they can *prevent* the development of chronic schizophrenia is more uncertain. Most clinicians who treat schizophrenia doubt that they do, but there are enthusiasts who think these drugs prevent chronic deterioration in at least some schizophrenics.

Neuroleptic drugs can prevent acute episodes if they are taken continuously, but the price for doing that is regarded as too high by many doctors and by almost all patients. Drugs used for schizophrenia are punishing to take, as George's course illustrates. In fact, it is sometimes hard to distinguish between chronic schizophrenia and the effects of the drugs used to treat acute schizophrenia. Patients experience lethargy and increased muscle tone, which produces an uncomfortable stiffness that makes movement labored. Often a tremor like that seen in Parkinson's disease is present. At the same time, those who are taking the drugs report "restless legs," a need to keep in motion. Although other medicines can help minimize discomforts due to the side effects, people taking neuroleptics just do not feel completely well. Doctors and their patients face a difficult trade-off: vulnerability to the major signs of illness versus discomfort from drugs. Doctors have tended to downplay the negative effects in favor of overtreatment, whereas most patients prefer to minimize the side effects and therefore to undertreat, taking their chances with the disease.

One long-term unwanted effect of the major tranquilizers is *tardive dyskinesia* (literally "late-appearing disordered movement"), which usually appears when the dose of the drug is reduced or stopped entirely. Tardive dyskinesia commonly consists of involuntary smacking or sucking movements of the lips or writhing movements of the tongue, but virtually the entire body may be involved. There is no pain or discomfort; the damage, which is often great, is to the social acceptability of the affected person. The movements are unpleasant to see. The only treatment is to re-establish the accustomed dose of drug. In some cases the disordered movements may decrease after months or years, but authorities consider most of the damage permanent. The risk increases with potency and dose of drugs: Potent drugs taken at high doses for long periods of time maximize the risk for tardive dyskinesia.

The best current practice is to treat schizophrenia with major tranquilizers when delusions, hallucinations, fragmented thinking, or some combination of the three is present. The dose should be the lowest consistent with suppression of those manifestations of illness. After suppression is accomplished, the dose should be continued for several weeks and then slowly reduced. This treatment may continue for some time—several months, perhaps—but eventually the drug should be completely withdrawn and not used further unless the disease flares up again.

A new drug, clozapine (Clozaril), which has just come onto the American market, seems to be having a profound beneficial effect on some persons with schizophrenia, including reversal of at least some features of chronic schizophrenia. Clozapine has a somewhat different mode of action from other neuroleptics, though one not completely defined. Like other drugs effective in schizophrenia, clozapine blocks dopamine receptors, but apparently not all of them, just a select population in one functional area of the brain (the limbic system). This may explain why, among its other virtues, it does not produce tardive dyskinesia—indeed, it may reduce it because the dopamine receptors implicated in that side effect are in another area (the striatum). Clozapine does have serious side effects, however; the most dangerous of these is suppression of the bone marrow's production of white blood cells, which has been fatal in some cases. It also induces epileptic seizures in some persons. For these reasons, clozapine is now given only to persons with severe schizophrenia who have not responded to other treatments. About 10 to 20 percent of those persons have improved so dramatically that new hope and enthusiasm are permeating treatment centers. Several other new drugs with similar modes of action are being developed in the hope of improving efficacy still further and reducing side effects, especially suppression of the bone marrow activity. The continuing development of these preparations, called *atypical antipsychotics* in the medical literature, promises enormous benefits to sufferers from a cruel disease.

As always, treatment with drugs must be combined with education and especially with vocational counseling. Every effort must be made to help the person with schizophrenia play a productive role in society for as long as possible. Although a few victims may not be able to work at all, many hold regular jobs indefinitely, and some do reasonably well in sheltered workshops. However, until better treatments are developed, many schizophrenics will be unable to function adequately as independent adults in families, much less in society. Such persons need asylum, and providing it was a major function of the state hospital of a few decades past. Box 2 describes one unintended effect of the dismantling of the state hospital system.

■ *If You Have Schizophrenia*

You have a serious disease, but better treatments are arriving. And, meanwhile, there are things that you should do for yourself in addition to learning everything you can about the disease and its treatment. "Street" drugs, including some (like marijuana) with benign reputations, seem to be especially hazardous for people with your illness. Avoid them. Perhaps most central to your illness, you must keep doing life's conventional things— working, making "small talk," doing household chores—even though you don't feel able. Yours is one of the few illness that requires that you do things *despite* how you feel. Finally, keep hope alive in yourself. If you have just developed the disease, it may turn out to be mild and give you little trouble through the rest of your life. If it is more severe, present treatments will help a lot, and the next generation of drugs now being developed holds realistic promise of keeping your illness in check indefinitely. Hang in there.

■ *If Someone Close to You Has Schizophrenia*

Schizophrenia is an especially difficult illness for families to deal with. One important reassurance: Relatives, especially parents, should realize that their rearing practices are not responsible for the disease. Blaming parents—usually the "schizophrenogenic (schizophrenia-causing) mother"—was once a fashionable dogma of "therapy" tendered by popular schools, but there is absolutely *no* evidence that actions of relatives cause the disease.

Box 2   Mental Illness and the Homeless

California, a typical state with respect to care of those suffering from mental illness, operates 5000 beds in state mental hospitals. There would be 50,000 beds if the state hospitals were occupied at California's 1960 rates. The incidence of psychiatric illness has not changed, so where are the 45,000 persons who are not occupying those beds? Many of them are not ill, or are not ill enough to need hospitalization, because treatments have improved. The members of another large group reside in halfway houses and various other room-and-board facilities supported by governments at all levels. These people are moderately to severely impaired. But these two groups do not account for the great majority of the people not occupying beds in California state hospitals. To see what has happened to the rest, one has only to walk the streets of any large American city. Many of these chronically mentally ill persons are living, and often dying, on the streets. About 80 percent of all the adult homeless have a chronic psychiatric illness; most exhibit schizophrenia or drug dependence. How to deal with this emerging tragedy poses immense problems for our society.

Homelessness is partly the unintended result of over-zealous protection of the "rights" of the mentally ill by the courts and the acceptance of easy answers by state legislatures. When George was first discharged from the hospital, responsibility for his treatment was transferred to a community mental health clinic. Started in the mid-1960s, these clinics were intended to provide treatment in their home communities for persons with mental handicaps. Some mental health professionals thought that this would minimize the role of state hospitals and state schools for the retarded, preventing "hospitalism" and "warehousing." This viewpoint found an eager audience. Congress appropriated funds needed to establish the centers, and the states, though at first resentful of federal leadership (which was seen as usurping their traditional role with respect to mental illness), soon joined the effort. Optimism nourished wholesome motives. Most of those concerned were appalled by the plight of the mentally ill and retarded. Moreover, they sincerely believed that mental illness was the product of the social environment and that a healthy society could take care of the problem—indeed, should be forced to take care of it. The community caused it; the community should deal with it. Political motivations were darker. State legislatures saw that transferring responsibility to communities from state institutions, mainly state hospitals, would shift fiscal responsibility to the federal welfare system. Moreover, reducing the populations of state institutions saved a lot of money. And closing facilities, when feasible, also made it possible to sell the large farms that most of the institutions owned, creating irresistible windfalls when budgets required balancing.

The community mental health movement has yielded mixed results. Despite the expectations of early enthusiasts, illness was not cured or prevented. However, providing treatment close to home in smaller, decentralized clinics was an excellent idea from which many patients and families benefited. The "downside" is that governments never provided funds to establish enough centers or to adequately staff those whicht were created. The centers limped along. Over the years, despite this halting start, some centers matured into highly responsible and effective organizations that provide quality treatment in humane settings. However, their most effective services have been focused on children and families, not on the severely ill, chronic patients they had been expected to serve.

Ironically, it was finding mentally ill persons housed in scattered county homes and room-and-board facilities in the centers of large cities that prompted Dorothea Dix to

(Continued)

(Box 2 continued)

lead the reform movement that produced the nation's state hospital system in the mid-nineteenth century. She saw that ill persons lacked adequate sanitation and medical care, and were vulnerable to exploitation by criminals. Dismayed, Dix persuaded the Massachusetts legislature to establish a state hospital system that became a model for the nation. Sadly, in important respects, we have come full circle.

This history strongly suggests that humane governments might best help persons such as George by both putting adequate resources into community mental health centers *and* resurrecting state hospital systems. Good community mental health centers have demonstrated that they can do an excellent job treating some of the chronically ill. But not all. We still need state hospitals of the type that a few decades ago furnished adequate medical care and reasonably clean and healthful living accommodations. The patients provided for many of their own needs; most of them worked on farms, in kitchens, or on the grounds. State hospitals were far from perfect, but they offered patients a degree of safety, humane care, and social usefulness that the current system does not provide. Before rejecting the paternalism implied by such a prescription, social theorists should look at the alternative provided by the streets.

Apart from resolving to remember this, the most helpful thing that families can do is to reduce the emotional level prevailing in the home. Research has established that a high level of "expressed emotion" is a most important factor leading to flare-ups of the disease. Persons with schizophrenia tolerate emotional display poorly. Families differ greatly in the degree of emotional volatility accepted as an intrinsic part of family life, but every family can tone it down somewhat. Here are the most useful steps:

- Try to minimize family criticism of the ill person. Do this by lowering expectations to correspond with the ill person's ability to comply. This is tricky. Be guided by experience, common sense, and professional advice.

- Avoid confrontations. Argue with other family members only when the ill person is not present.

- Don't get overinvolved with the ill person, and don't smother him or her with emotional support. On the contrary, give less than your inclinations suggest. Allow emotional distance.

- Establish predictable routines. Have meals and other family activities at the same time each day. In this regard, it will be most helpful to schedule daily activities for the ill person. A regular job is best, but a sheltered workshop or day hospital is also well worth finding.

- Minimize contact with relatives and friends who have emotionally reactive or evocative personalities.

Fitting any of these recommendations to a specific family is difficult. And although mild to moderate illness may be kept within manageable limits, severely ill persons can so dominate a household that life for others, especially young siblings, is distorted beyond reason. Be sure that other family members have outlets outside the home, and don't allow the family to withdraw from friends and relatives. If the ill person cannot be maintained at home, local social agencies will be able to tell you about acceptable alternatives, such as board-and-care houses. And finally, remember that promising new treatments are being developed, even for severe disease.

Schizoid Disorders

Many relatives of schizophrenics seem eccentric or disturbed in ways that recall schizophrenia, especially in their emotional coldness and anhedonia. These conditions have been called *schizoid*

Box 3 Does Mental Illness Run in Families?

Yes it does. Moreover, enough studies of adopted children
and other special populations have been done to convince
most authorities that genes go further than disturbed family environment toward accounting for the relationship.
The implications of these findings will be discussed in
chapters to come. But in the meantime, we should note the
key role that studies of diseases within families have
played in the development of psychiatry.

Much of the foundation for modern psychiatry was
laid in Munich, Germany, from about 1890 to 1925.
Pioneering psychiatrists began with virtually no criteria for
distinguishing among the different types of mental disease:
They had no bases for diagnosis. Fully aware that that
diagnosis was essential because it implied a prognosis,
they studied the natural history of illnesses in order to
develop syndromes analogous to those of general
medicine. Which clusters of signs and symptoms remained
constant from one episode of illness to the next? Which
predicted recovery and which deterioration?

Family studies provided crucial evidence. These
early psychiatrists were sure that coincidence could not
explain the large numbers of abnormal persons in the

(schizophrenia-like) *disorders* or *schizophrenic spectrum disorders*.
Their relationship to schizophrenia is unclear and is a subject of
debate among specialists. An historical perspective on this and
analogous problems with other diseases is presented in Box 3. This
will help in understanding the puzzles these disorders present to
psychiatry today.

Most of the relatives of schizophrenics who are disturbed, exhibit disturbances of behavior and personality that resemble a mild
form of chronic schizophrenia. However, not only is the disability

families of their patients. Illnesses that were found to be concentrated within families probably shared common causal factors, whereas conditions not so concentrated did not. For example, relatives of schizophrenics were at high risk for schizophrenia or a schizoid disorder, but *not* at high risk for bipolar illness, or obsessional illness, or alcoholism, or epilepsy. This made it reasonably certain that the latter conditions were not related to schizophrenia. Moreover, similar patterns were found for nearly all of the other illnesses to be described in the following chapters. Most often these patterns made intuitive sense. For example, cyclothymic personalities were found in families in which other members had bipolar illness. But sometimes the patterns were counterintuitive: A concentration of alcoholics was found in families in which others suffered from depression. The syndromes so developed have largely withstood repeated attempts to refine, modify, or repeal them, and today they are still firmly in place. However, several "loose ends" remain. An important theme of this book will be describing, and trying to account for, the concentrations of disorders found in families marked by psychiatric illness.

relatively slight, but such persons also do not exhibit the hallucinations and flagrantly disturbed thinking of acute schizophrenia.

Paranoid disorders constitute a large subgroup of schizoid disorders and provide a useful illustration of them, including the fact that their status is shaky—starting with nomenclature. Paranoid disorders have also been known as paranoia, paranoid state, and late-onset paraphrenia. (The diversity of labels underscores the lack of agreement among experts about their place among the mental illnesses.)

Paranoid disorders are marked by suspiciousness and delusions, and, especially because of the delusions, they resemble schizophrenia. This seems fitting, as these disorders do distinguish some relatives of schizophrenics. However, only some persons with a paranoid disorder have any apparent connection to schizophrenia. The genealogical connection is only a weak clue. Paranoid disorders become more frequent with age. The associated delusions are as uncorrectable as any, and they can be so intense and disabling that some authorities regard paranoid disorders as simply late-onset schizophrenia. However, the delusions tend to be relatively well organized in that they often revolve around specific themes. And unlike persons with typical schizophrenia, those affected deal rationally—often very competently—with other aspects of life.

One common theme of the delusions is jealousy. The result of such delusions is often called *jealousy paranoia,* a condition that begins with the absolute conviction that the affected person's spouse is unfaithful. Any observation, no matter how irrelevant or trivial, may be distorted to support the conviction. A present from the spouse is merely a crude attempt to divert attention from an affair being carried on with a neighbor. Attentiveness to a spouse at a party is a sham to hide signals being exchanged between spouse and lover. He bought himself a new necktie. We know whom he is trying to impress. And what happened to the tie he had on when he left home? After an especially good night's sleep, one affected husband noted that the guest bedroom was in slight disarray. Obviously, he had been drugged so that his wife could entertain.

There are no specific treatments for these disorders, which tend to be very stable once established, getting neither better nor worse. Drugs used in schizophrenia sedate and so dampen problematic behavior, but they are not otherwise effective.

Chapter

4

Alzheimer's Disease and Other Dementing Illnesses

□ □ □

❏ *Harry*

Harry appeared to be in perfect health at age 58, except that for a few days he had had a nasty flu. He worked in the municipal water treatment plant of a small city, and it was at work that the first overt signs of Harry's mental illness appeared. While responding to a minor emergency, he became confused about the correct order in which to pull the levers that controlled the flow of fluids. As a result, several thousand gallons of raw sewage were discharged into a river. Harry had been an efficient and diligent worker, so after puzzled questioning, his error was attributed to the flu and overlooked.

Several weeks later, Harry came home with a baking dish his wife had asked him to buy, having forgotten that he had brought home the identical dish two nights before. Later that week, on two successive nights, he went to pick up his daughter at her job

87

in a restaurant, apparently forgetting that she had changed shifts and was now working days. A month after that, he quite uncharacteristically argued with a clerk at the phone company; he was trying to pay a bill that he had already paid three days before.

By this time his wife had become alarmed about the changes in Harry. Thinking back, she began to piece together episodes that convinced her that his memory had actually been undependable for at least several months, perhaps much longer. When she discovered that he had been writing reminder notes to himself on odd scraps of paper and that these included detailed instructions about how to operate machinery at work if various problems arose, she insisted that he see a doctor. He himself realized that his memory had been failing, and so he agreed with his wife, though reluctantly. The doctor did a physical examination and ordered several laboratory tests, including an electroencephalogram (a brain wave test). The examination results were normal, and the doctor thought the problem might be depression. He prescribed an antidepressant drug, but if anything, it seemed to make Harry's memory worse. It certainly did not make him feel any better. That treatment failing, the doctor thought that Harry must have hardening of the arteries of the brain, about which, he said, nothing could be done.

Months passed and Harry's wife was beside herself. She could see that his problem was worsening. Not only had she been unable to get effective help, but Harry himself was becoming resentful and sometimes suspicious of her attempts. He now insisted there was nothing wrong with him, and she would catch him narrowly watching her every movement. From time to time he accused her of having the police watch him, and he would draw all the blinds in the house. Once he ripped the telephone out of the wall, convinced it was "spying." Sometimes he became angry—sudden little storms without apparent cause. He would shout angrily at his wife and occasionally throw or kick things. Such episodes did not seem dangerous because they were short-lived and because Harry seemed more frustrated than angry. His outbursts lacked sustained direction and intensity. More difficult for his wife was Harry's repetitiveness in conversation: He often repeated stories from the past and sometimes repeated isolated phrases and sentences from more recent exchanges. There was no context and little continuity to his choice of subjects. He might recite the same story or instruction several times a day. His work was also a great cause of deep concern. His wife, who had the summer off from her position as a fourth-grade teacher, began checking on him at his job at least once a day. Soon she was actually doing most of his work. His supervisor, an old friend of the family, looked the other way. Harry seemed grateful that his wife was there.

Two years after Harry had first allowed the sewage to escape, he was clearly a changed man. Most of the time he seemed preoccupied; he usually had a vacant smile on his face, and what little he said was so vague that it lacked meaning. He had entirely given up his main interests (golf and woodworking), and he became careless about his person. More and more, for example, he slept in his clothes. Gradually his wife took over getting him up, toileted, and dressed each morning.

One day the county supervisor stopped by to tell his wife that Harry just could not work any longer. A disability insurance policy would carry him for the few months until he was 62, and then he would be eligible for early retirement. He hadn't really worked for a long while anyway, and he had become so inattentive that he had to be kept away from machinery. He was just too much of a burden on his co-workers. Harry himself still insisted that nothing was wrong, but by now no one tried to explain things to him. He had long since stopped reading. His days were spent sitting vacantly in front of the television, but he couldn't describe any of the programs he had watched.

Harry's condition continued to worsen slowly. When his wife's school was in session, his daughter would stay with him some days, and neighbors were able to offer some help. But occasionally he would still manage to wander away. On those occasions he greeted everyone he met—old friends and strangers alike—with "Hi, it's so nice." That was the extent of his conversation, although he might repeat "nice, nice, nice" over and over again. He had promised not to drive, but one day he did take the family automobile and promptly got lost. The police brought him home, and his wife took the car keys and kept them. When Harry left a coffee pot on a unit of the electric stove until it melted, his wife, desperate for help, took him to see another doctor. Again Harry was found to be in good health. This time the doctor ordered a *CAT scan* (*c*omputed *a*xial *t*omography), a sophisticated X-ray examination that made a visual image of Harry's brain, which, it revealed, had actually shrunk in size. The doctor said that Harry had "Pick-Alzheimer disease" and that there was no known cause and no effective treatment.

Harry could no longer be left at home alone, so his daughter began working nights and caring for him until his wife came home after school. He would sit all day, except that sometimes he would wander aimlessly through the house. Safety latches at each entrance kept him from going outdoors, though he no longer seemed interested in that—or in much of anything else. He had no memory for events of the day and little recollection of occasions from the distant past, which a year or so before he had enjoyed describing. His speech consisted of repeating the same word or phrase over and over (for example, "Hooky then, hooky then, hooky then"). His wife kept trying to find help. She inquired at the state mental hospitals but was told that because Harry wasn't dangerous, he was not eligible for admission.

Because Harry was a veteran, she took him to the nearest Veterans Administration Hospital, which was 150 miles away. After a stay of nine weeks, during which the CAT scan and all the other tests were repeated with the same results, the doctors said Harry had a chronic brain syndrome. They advised long-term hospitalization in a regional veterans' hospital about 400 miles away from his home. Meanwhile his wife, who wanted Harry closer to home, had found that local nursing homes would charge more than her monthly take-home pay to care for him and that Medicare would not pay nursing home charges. Desperate, five years after the accident at work, she accepted with gratitude hospitalization at the veterans' hospital so far away.

At the hospital the nursing staff sat Harry up in a chair each day and, aided by volunteers, made sure he ate enough. Still, he lost weight and became weaker. He would weep when his wife came to see him, but he did not talk, and he gave no other sign that he recognized her. After a year, even the weeping stopped. Harry's wife could no longer bear to visit. Harry lived on until just after his sixty-fifth birthday, when he choked on a piece of bread, developed pneumonia as a consequence, and soon died.

Diagnosis: Alzheimer's Disease

Harry had Alzheimer's disease, although this diagnosis was not definitively established until after his death, when an autopsy was done. Alzheimer's disease is not the only disease that can produce the signs and symptoms of illness that Harry exhibited, but it is the most common; about 70 percent of people with Harry's signs and symptoms turn out to have Alzheimer's disease. Among the other *dementing illnesses,* or dementias, the main one is Pick's disease. These diseases impose an enormous burden on our society—one that will increase as our population ages. They begin to affect appreciable numbers of people starting at about age 50, and their frequency increases with age until by about age 85, between 20 and 30 percent of all people who reach that age will be affected. Males and females are at equal risk, but more females are affected because as a group they live longer.

Unfortunately, these diseases cannot be separated one from another without an autopsy. The diagnosis of Alzheimer's disease is made by a neuropathologist, who finds in brain tissue characteristic microscopic changes called *neurofibrillary tangles* and *senile plaques.* These changes occur in or around neurons, the working cells of the brain. They may occur in most parts of the brain, but they are present in greatest numbers in areas most directly involved with memory and higher intellectual function. Whereas demonstrable chemical abnormalities characterize other illnesses described in this book, in Alzheimer's disease, brain tissue can actually be seen to be diseased.

Diseased nerve cells no longer function properly. From nerve cells come the commands that set our muscles into motion. These cells also contain our memories, receive the sights and sounds by which we know our surroundings, and cause our hormones to be secreted. They *are* mood and affect—our emotions. They constitute the physical basis of what we call mind. Nerve cells involved with the plaques and tangles of Alzheimer's disease look dead. Obviously, a brain containing many of them is not functioning well enough to interpret life in all its richness or to mount human responses to it. That is what happened to Harry.

Over the past decade, much has been learned about the biology of Alzheimer's disease. The nerve cells that are lost originate from a small area at the base of the brain. Acetylcholine is their neurotransmitter, so their loss results in a deficit in choline acetyl transferase, the enzyme needed to join acetyl to choline. There are deficits in other neurotransmitters, but insufficient acetylcholine is the most prominent and the most consistently found. Several attempts at treatment have been based on supplying the brain with more acetylcholine or preventing its destruction in the synaptic cleft (see Figure 1). None of these attempts has succeeded yet, but the strategy makes sense and the search continues.

A strange coincidence led to another advance. People with Down's syndrome develop the same changes in brain tissue—plaques, tangles, and lack of acetylcholine—that are found in Alzheimer's disease. These changes apparently occur in all people with Down's syndrome, and they occur by age 40—much earlier in life than in Alzheimer's disease. Down's is caused by an extra copy of chromosome 21, so this clue has led Alzheimer's researchers to that chromosome. Their efforts have led to a much deeper understanding of the biology of Alzheimer's disease. Describing this would take us too far into highly technical material to be useful, but Chapter 10 presents an overview of the rationale undergirding current brain research and the remarkable progress being made.

Signs and Symptoms

Memory Loss

Memory loss is the central feature of Alzheimer's disease and similar illnesses. To understand the signs and symptoms of these illnesses, it is important to recognize the distinction between *short-term*, or *immediate*, *memory*, and *long-term*, or *distant*, *memory*. In our short-term memory we retain enough information about our immediate environment and its very recent history to enable us to monitor it continuously and adjust our responses accordingly. This memory tells us where we parked our automobile. However, we remember little of this material very long. Why should we? This information would be most unlikely to have value for us, and there must be some limit to our storage capacity. For example, we can usually (although perhaps with effort) recall where we parked in the supermarket lot the day before yesterday. We are unlikely to remember much of anything about the shopping trip before that one.

Although quite a lot is known about conditions that promote or inhibit long-term memory formation, the exact mechanisms are among the major unsolved problems of neuroscience. What we do eventually store in long-term memory is first established as short-term memory, but then other brain mechanisms must become involved. We can establish long-term memory by consciously deciding to remember and then making a special effort. For example, if we make an extraordinary effort, we can memorize nonsense symbols and retain them in memory indefinitely. We can remember important facts for long periods, and our memory is enhanced if we occasionally recall and use these facts. (Retention of the vocabulary of a foreign language provides a good example of this process.) Events that produce an emotional response may remain in our memory whether we want them there or not. As it happens, I was eating lunch when I heard that President Kennedy had been assassinated. I remember quite vividly that I was in a hospital cafeteria, eating a hamburger, and sitting with two colleagues whose faces I can still see and whose names I still recall. Affective responses, positive or negative, engage powerful learning mechanisms.

The first sign of dementing illness is nearly always the loss of recent memories—and the resulting failure to create new long-term memories. However, immediate recall is often normal. An example will make these distinctions clear. In a bedside test frequently used by professionals, a patient is asked to remember the names of five common objects chosen by the examiner and then to repeat them (1) immediately after they are presented and (2) after a delay of a minute or two. The normal response is to repeat correctly four or five of the names both immediately and after one or two minutes. If anything, the performance of normal people improves after the delay. The performance of patients with even early dementia, however, usually declines after the delay. They typically will repeat four or five names immediately but can recall only one or two after the delay.

Material already established in long-term memory tends to be preserved much longer in people with dementia. The result is that a person who cannot retain enough recent information to count change may recall a wedding or high school football game in vivid detail. The same person may remember an emotionally charged event of a month before but be unable to converse about events that took place that day. Eventually, as the disease progresses, long-term memory fails as well.

Harry's history illustrates the importance of the distinction between immediate and long-term memory. He could manage routine operations on his job, but when he had to deal with a minor emergency that required enough recent memory for him to function effectively while deviating from routine, his disability became evident. Likewise, he managed to pick up his daughter from at her job as long as doing so was a nightly routine. When the routine changed, Harry failed to adapt.

Harry's history also illustrates a concept that is most important in medicine, the *threshold*. It is not unusual for a major illness apparently to begin with a minor one. Our organ systems, including our brains, have reserve capacities beyond those needed to cope with life's ordinary demands. If that reserve capacity is gradually lost to disease, the loss may go unnoticed until an added stress, such as Harry's flu, makes demands on the system that cannot be met. Then what had been an adequate—though marginal—adaptation may suddenly be lost. This can be quite confusing to people close to someone who develops a major illness. We naturally try to attach a cause to an illness, too often wrongly assuming or assigning guilt: "If only I hadn't made him go out in the rain" or "Our son was such a worry to him." We seek understandable explanations and too easily accept the one that seems most immediate. We are usually wrong. Meeting challenges to one's physical capacities is an ordinary part of life. We cannot avoid acknowledging disease by pretending that the challenge caused the problem.

Impaired Judgment

Next to loss of recent memory, the most noticeable defect in dementia, as it progresses, is diminution of the logical and social capacities that we call judgment. We all continually respond to challenges from our environment, which require that we obtain information, integrate it into our consciousness, and make responses or choose not to respond. We thus exercise judgment.

Dementing people are not able to assimilate information so efficiently as they did before becoming ill, and therefore their responses are less adept. At first the deficits may be noticeable only in the nuances of social deportment. For example, the dementing person may become uncharacteristically inattentive to conversation. The whole context of social situations is not grasped as before, and the quality of responses declines as a result. However, long-established patterns of behavior that have become more or less automatic tend to be preserved. It is the dementing person's response to new situations, new people, new facts, and new environments that makes the developing disability evident.

Abstraction

Closely related to judgment is the ability to abstract, and this capacity too declines in dementia. Finding common themes and sorting important from unimportant details requires this ability. The loss can be difficult to detect in one who has spent a lifetime dealing with abstract ideas. The same words and phrases are used that served well before illness developed, and they may sound superficially convincing. Only close examination may reveal the underlying vagueness and poverty of thought. A common test is to ask a patient to name as many four-footed animals as he or she can. The normal response is to use groups to organize the effort: cows, horses, pigs, etc. (barnyard animals); lions, zebras, elephants, etc. (African wild animals); and so on. Even moderate dementia interferes with this process. Fewer animals are named, and grouping is not so evident: lions, pigs, mice, and so on.

Emotionality

Changes in emotional responsiveness occur, usually after the loss of memory has become evident. Early in the course, a general decrease in responsiveness may coexist with rare episodes of heightened responsiveness that are often quite alien to the previous personality. Hypersexuality, coarsening of humor, irritability, and sometimes physical striking out may appear. Later, as the disease progresses, apathy and uninvolvement come to dominate.

Harry's behaviors were typical. He attempted to hide his growing disability by writing little notes to spur his memory. Early in the course of his illness, he exhibited some emotional unevenness, especially temper outbursts, that were short-lived and not really targeted. Underlying these changes in behavior, Harry became more suspicious and generally paranoid in his outlook. This is a fairly common development in dementia. It can be quite troublesome, but in most cases the erroneous ideas and unfounded suspicions are held only briefly and do not seem to generate much emotional fervor. Later Harry became totally unresponsive. In retrospect, it is clear that the changes in Harry's behavior marked unmistakable and irreversible stages in the destruction of his brain and, with it, his personality.

Prognosis

The diseases that cause dementia progress at a fairly steady rate that is unrelieved by periods of improvement. This is an important distinguishing characteristic. Many illnesses impair memory, and a slow, very gradual decline in memory called *benign senescent forgetfulness* is associated with normal aging. But such conditions do not produce the inexorable progression of memory loss seen in Alzheimer's disease and similar dementing illnesses. Even though true dementing illnesses may seem to progress little, or not at all, over fairly extended periods, studies of brain metabolism reveal a linear and inexorable decline in function. Periods with no apparent progression are merely periods between thresholds. Later in the course, more remote memories begin to fade. The affected person may recall events long past, but his or her descriptions become poorer in details. Later still, as in Harry's case, the victim does not recognize members of the immediate family. Communication of any kind becomes rare, and toward the end it effectively ceases.

The affected person becomes less physically active. More time is spent staring off into space. Later in the course, there may be changes in the nervous control of muscles. These changes most often produce rigidity due to increased muscle tone (hypertonicity). Because of this rigidity, the dementing person may need help bringing food to his or her mouth. Rigidity may also produce painful cramping, which is often especially troublesome at night. Eventually the illness advances until the affected person is bedfast.

Seizures (epileptic fits) may also develop late in the course. These usually take the form of rapid alternating movements of arms or legs, or both. Seizures are alarming to those unaccustomed to seeing them. However, they are usually quite harmless when they appear as a feature of dementing illness, and to the ill person, they are less distressing than cramps.

Just before the last stages are reached, there is often a substantial loss of weight. Most affected persons have to be fed. If loss of control of bladder and bowel has not occurred during the previous months, it certainly occurs at this time. Skilled nursing care is generally required to prevent bed sores from becoming a major problem. Death, which comes 8 to 12 years after onset, is not directly due to brain disease. Rather, the victim succumbs to some incidental event: pneumonia, strokes, kidney infection, or choking on food. The real cause is one of the cruelest diseases to assail the human spirit.

Other Dementing Illnesses

Several other diseases have much the same effects as Alzheimer's disease. Two of the most distinctive are Huntington's disease and Pick's disease.

Huntington's Disease

This illness is characterized by peculiar writhing movements first of the extremities and later (often) of the whole body. In about half of the cases, however, the first sign is a psychiatric illness—usually mania or depression, less often a paranoid state. Huntington's is a rare disease affecting only 5 of every 100,000 adults in the general population. The average age at onset is about 42 and the disease progresses to death over 12 to 15 years. Huntington's disease is genetically inherited as an autosomal dominant trait, which means that on average, 50 percent of the parents, siblings, and children of an affected person are themselves affected and that females and males are at equal risk. (The implications of this genetic relationship will be discussed in the last section of this book.)

Pick's Disease

Most cases of this disease are indistinguishable from Alzheimer's disease unless an autopsy is done. However, a few Pick's cases do exhibit a peculiar syndrome, the most noticeable feature of which is gross overeating. Large weight gains may occur, and patients have been known to choke to death on food or on other things, such as toilet paper, that they have stuffed in their mouth. The average age at onset is 54 years, and the average time until death—8 years—is relatively short.

Treatment

No treatment of the basic disease process has yet been proved effective—or even promising—for any of the dementias. There is no known way to slow the progression of the disease, much less stop it. Yet there is a great deal that can be done to minimize the human suffering produced. Some especially strong or fortunate families even seem to thrive despite the terrible adversity of dementing illness. The following are commonsense suggestions based on my experience.

■   *If You Suspect You Have a Dementing Illness*

First, beware of self-diagnosis. We all forget, and most of us are quick to become alarmed by our lapses. Most often the cause is simple human fallibility, and sometimes a common disease such as depression is at fault. Do not assume that you have an irreversible dementing illness. If you are sure your memory is getting worse, see a doctor for a competent diagnosis.

If the presence of dementing illness is confirmed, the prognosis is poor but there is reason to hope. Some 15 drug preparations aimed at correcting the known biochemical defect in Alzheimer's disease are being tested in major medical centers. Also, for two decades researchers have been puzzled by inconclusive hints that aluminum concentrations in brain may be minutely increased in Alzheimer's disease. Simple environmental exposure to aluminum does not explain this finding because smelter workers and persons who have taken medications containing aluminum for decades do not develop Alzheimer's disease at excessive rates. However, it is possible that a genetic vulnerability (as will be explained in Chapter 10) may cause some persons to have impaired ability to dispose of aluminum that reaches their tissues. And aluminum is one of the most abundant elements, so some considerable exposure is inevitable. Based on this research, a 1991 report described an attempt at chelation therapy in persons with clinically diagnosed Alzheimer's disease (no autopsies). Chelation removes metallic elements such as aluminum from tissue. The result was that the treatment appeared to slow the progression of the dementing process. Slowing the progression of a dementing disease is extremely difficult to demonstrate, and more studies with large numbers of subjects will be required before this hopeful result can be confirmed. Studies of treatment using chelation or other drugs are ongoing at many medical centers. Inquire at your local chapter of the Alzheimer's Association about studies in your area and volunteer for one; you'll learn a lot and make an important contribution.

Try to live within your capabilities. Limit your physical horizon. Draw your boundaries according to where you feel perfectly comfortable; keep your excursions within your neighborhood, your block, your yard. You will continue to find pleasure in life's ordinary events. Savor them and focus on them; live a day at a time.

■ *If Someone Close to You Has Alzheimer's Disease or Another Dementia*

Try always to keep the nature of the disability in mind. The main problem is with memory. Three common impediments to memory are encountered in everyday life. They are not often important to a normal brain, but they can compromise an impaired one. Minimizing them can help. The first of these is fatigue. People with brain impairment are nearly always at their best after a period of rest. Schedule strenuous events such as a visit to the doctor after a period of sleep. Encourage naps.

The second major impediment to memory is anxiety. Anxiety powerfully interferes with memory formation. A vicious circle can be set up in which memory failure results in lack of ability to respond to environmental challenges. This increases anxiety, which further impairs memory, and so on. Use anxiety as a signal. When signs of anxiety appear, say at a social gathering, it is time to leave. Nothing will effectively relieve the anxiety except removal from the difficult situation.

The third major impediment is drugs. Unfortunately, all drugs that are classified as sedatives interfere with memory. These drugs include alcohol, Valium and related drugs, and barbiturates. Be aware what drugs are being used, and note their effect.

In addition to watching out for hazards, there are positive things you can do. Get good at reorienting the person you are caring for by compensating for his or her memory with your own. A typical example might arise from the grandchildren's visit. Suppose that they are playing in the next room, from whence you hear a sudden noise. The healthy brain remembers instantly: "Oh, the children are in the next room; that explains the noise. It doesn't sound dangerous, they're just playing." But for the brain that cannot remember what is going on in the next room, such sudden noises are unaccountable and so cause alarm and anxiety. Being aware of this, upon hearing the noise you simply say softly, "That is the children playing in the next room. They are O.K."

Social occasions can be difficult. Keep the numbers of new faces and new names to a minimum. Social conversations tend to focus on current events, the dementing person's weakest point. Help by judiciously supplying answers and steering conversation toward safer topics. Or reminisce unabashedly. Again, most of all, be aware of developing anxiety. Virtually any sign of discomfort is a signal that capacity is at or approaching overload.

Guard against overestimating the victim's mental capacity, a much more common error than underestimating it. Remember that capacity varies through the day and is especially vulnerable to fatigue. Dementing persons, like the rest of us, try hard to perform the best they can. Think twice when you are tempted to attribute a failure to willful lack of effort. Also, contrary to much well-meant advice, exercising the brain does *not* improve or preserve functional capacities. The brain is not a muscle and is quite unlike one in this respect.

Be matter-of-fact in conversation. Avoid ambiguity, and do not present unnecessary choices or decisions. Say "Now we must go to the store," not "Would you like to come to the store with me?" Be concrete: "Alan is coming to visit after lunch," not "We are going to have company today." Give positive directions: "Now it is time to take a shower," not "Shall we eat now, or would you rather shower first?"

Sometimes sedation is needed during the course of a dementing illness. Aggressive behavior is not often a problem in dementia, and if it occurs, it usually lasts only a short time during the early stages of the illness. Agitation and insomnia are much more common, and sometimes administering medications is the only effective response. But there are trade-offs to consider. As noted earlier, any sedative drug interferes with memory. Major tranquilizers (neuroleptic drugs) may be a better answer, but they must be used carefully, because dementing persons are often exquisitely sensitive to them. Oversedation to the point of stupor, and very severe neuromuscular reactions like those George experienced, are particular hazards. If these drugs are needed, starting doses should be minute and any increases made gradually. A common first dose might be 1 milligram of a potent drug such as haloperidol.

Older persons excrete or destroy most drugs slower than younger persons. Therefore, drugs may accumulate longer in the body of an older person and thus reach higher concentrations for a given dose. Instead of a couple of days, it may take an older person a week before administered drugs reach equilibrium, the point at which the amount of drug excreted or destroyed equals the daily intake, producing a constant level in the blood. Through the period when blood levels are rising, excessive dosage may not be apparent, and then, when toxicity appears, it takes longer for blood levels to decrease. Remember that most often, sedation is needed only intermittently. Don't keep giving drugs as a matter of routine; rather, try reducing the dose whenever feasible. Learn from the prescribing doctor and your own experience what positive and negative effects to expect.

Dementing illness spawns immensely taxing medical, legal, social, and financial problems. Don't try to go it alone. There is an especially effective support group available to you in nearly all parts of the country, the Alzheimer's Association. Instructions for contacting it are given in Appendix B.

Part

3

ANXIETY

∎∎∎

ANXIETY is a feeling state, an affect. It is closely related to fear, except that anxiety is experienced when there is no apparent reason for fear. It is a physiologic response that is not under conscious control. We all know anxiety as a sporadic distress of everyday life. Nearly all psychiatric illnesses are accompanied by increased anxiety, but prolonged anxiety is the overriding feature of the illnesses described in this section. These are the *anxiety disorders*, formerly known as *neuroses*.

The word *anxiety* is descended from the Latin *angere*, which means "to choke or strangle." Breathlessness, often described as a feeling of suffocation or choking, is a common feature of anxiety. Other characteristic features include tremors, rapid and irregular heart action, chest pain, dizziness, sweating, nausea, abdominal cramps, diarrhea, and frequent urination.

Because anxiety blocks rational thought and impairs memory, it generates vicious circles: Inability to think clearly or remember

103

makes it difficult to manage problems, which in turn leads to greater anxiety. Anxiety also wastes energy; unproductive tension and agitation can cause intense fatigue.

Anxiety is helpful—even essential to survival—when it is associated with some actual or potential danger. Physical capacity is increased, preparing the body for fight or flight. Anxiety engages our most powerful learning mechanisms. Once anxiety becomes associated with a specific stimulus, we avoid that stimulus at almost any cost. In this way, we (and most animals) learn to avoid danger. We inhibit behavior that endangers us and become attentive to clues suggesting possible danger. At more humdrum levels, anxiety also motivates constructively. We feel a little restless, so we seek a safe place, prepare food, or clean our quarters. We are alert when crossing the street.

But anxiety-producing mechanisms are so easily activated that they sometimes punish even the most stoic among us. Think of some time when you faced an apparently hopeless problem. The world seemed to close in, and, miserable with apprehension and sick in your bowels, you paced about unable to rest, much less to act constructively. The feeling probably did not last long if you could do anything to stop it; we take almost any "out" because escaping anxiety is a most powerful motivator. If no escape is available, we do *something*, even if it is only pace the floor.

People with anxiety disorders experience such feelings throughout many of their waking hours and often through the hours normally reserved for sleep. They fully realize that there is no rational cause for the anxiety they feel—no threat, no danger. There is only extreme, irrational dis-ease.

Modern diagnosis recognizes seven variants of anxiety disorders: obsessive-compulsive disorder (also known as obsessional illness), post-traumatic stress disorder, panic disorder, simple phobia, social phobia, agoraphobia, and generalized anxiety disorder. As a rule, the first two of these are readily distinguished from the others. The last five are hard to separate from one another by any of the criteria generally used to delimit illnesses: They are much the same in signs, symptoms, course, and prognosis. Chapter 5 opens with a discussion of obsessive-compulsive disorder—a most distinctive condition—and then covers the other major anxiety disorders.

Chapter

5

Anxiety Disorders
□ □ □

❑ *Jerry*

Jerry was struggling. His rational, thinking self was pitted against an irrational, disgusting fear that he had gotten germs on the leg of the pants he was wearing. An hour before, during a rare venture out of his apartment to buy groceries, he had seen a woman walking a dog half a block in front of him. Just then he had happened to glance down. There, on a decorative wrought iron fence surrounding a tree, he saw a moist area where the dog might have urinated. The moisture was close to the right leg of his pants, but he saw immediately, to his great relief, that he was so far from the fence that his pants could not have touched the moist spot. He walked on. However, a few steps later, familiar doubts began. His leg had been parallel to the spot when he first noticed it. Perhaps he had swayed. Perhaps some urine had splattered to the sidewalk where he had walked. Perhaps a breeze

105

had carried his pant leg to the moisture. By the time he had finished his errands and returned to his apartment, the doubts were tormenting him. But he still felt in control.

Over the next hour, Jerry summoned all his rational arguments. He knew that his pant leg had not touched the urine. And what if it had? He had read that urine was sterile; it contained no germs. He also knew that germs were everywhere, that he couldn't possibly avoid them, and that even if he had touched the urine, it couldn't possibly harm him. He accepted all these arguments and marshaled many more, yet his discomfort increased. He felt unbearably restless. His stomach churned, he was gasping but still couldn't seem to get enough air, and his heart was pounding. He fought valiantly, tears in his eyes. But within the hour he had begun performing the ritual that would lead to putting the pants into his washer and bring him blessed—though only partial and temporary—relief.

The pants had to be cleaned in a special way. If the least detail were omitted, not only would the whole routine have to be repeated but other cleaning tasks would also be required. Jerry dreaded the prospect. More than once he had had to stay up cleaning all night, through the next day, and into the next night, until he collapsed from fatigue. Even after such an episode, he could not sleep in his bed if it were still "contaminated." He might have to sleep on the bare floor of his apartment.

Jerry stood on a plain stainless steel stool, untied his belt, and with exquisite care, slowly removed the pants. Great care was needed because he would have to clean anything that touched the pants. Of course he would have to wash his hands, his leg, his socks, his shoe, the stool, and the floor of the room. But there could well be more. Because he dreaded this, he had been extremely careful when he entered his apartment. He knew that he had not allowed his pants to touch his door jamb or brush against anything else. But he was again beset by doubts, and the questions were terribly insistent. Perhaps his pants had just barely touched the door. Perhaps a jet of air caused by opening the door had blown germs onto it. If he felt any doubt at all, he would have to clean the door and then everywhere that he had walked in the apartment. (He was meticulous about his budget too. During the last month he had spent $183.22 on cleaning materials.)

This time, Jerry almost got off lightly. He got the pants into the washer, with just the precise measures of detergent and bleach, that his ritual demanded, and the pants had touched nothing except his hands. Then he placed the other clothes he was wearing, including his shoes, in one side of his double, stainless-steel kitchen sink and got into the shower. He scrubbed every part of his body with a disposable brush, washing his hands exactly eighteen times according to a minutely prescribed routine. Starting at the shower, he scrubbed the floor with a new brush, working to the metal stool, which he picked up and took back to the shower. There he urinated (because he could urinate only in the shower, combining this necessity with cleaning saved time). Then he scrubbed the stool and scrubbed himself again, exactly as before. He dried himself very carefully, because any spot of water that fell from his body might be contaminated. Finally, he threw the towel into the kitchen sink on top of his other clothing. Lucky toss! It landed atop the clothing, touching nothing else. He filled the kitchen sink with water, measured in exactly the right amounts of detergent and disinfectant, and left the clothing to soak. By this time, Jerry was feeling almost normal. At least the unbearable tension was relieved.

His relief was short-lived. The telephone rang; his sister wanted to chat. At first he welcomed the call. Although Jerry saw his family only on important holidays and family occasions, the telephone kept them a close-knit group. His family had learned not to talk about Jerry's "cleaning binges" and other peculiarities. For his part, he knew that though they tried very hard to understand him, they just couldn't. He knew their arguments all too well: "You even admit you know it's just plain crazy to stand up for hours because you imagine that the seat of every chair is contaminated. So why do you do it to yourself?" In fact, he had often enough forced himself to sit in a "contaminated" chair. Sometimes a social situation demanded this of him. Other times he simply forced himself to behave rationally. His family couldn't understand him, but they didn't have to do the cleaning afterward.

"Hello, Jerry," his sister said. "What have you been up to? Making any money? You know, that electronic stock hit 47 today. Should I sell?" Jerry stumbled through a short conversation, all the while feeling the tension rising again. That number, 47, was a forbidden one. It was a prime number, and if he allowed its partner, 54, to enter his head, or if it came up in any way in conversation, the tension would increase unbearably. As the social exchange continued, he happened to notice a thick magazine, which he knew must contain a page 54. He couldn't possibly ignore or deny the fact of the magazine, and 47 plus 54 added up to 101. A prime number plus any other number that totaled 101 always meant fecal contamination. Bizarre, hopelessly bizarre, he realized. But he knew there was only one way to relieve the tension. After his sister hung up, he spent the next nine hours cleaning.

Jerry was fortunate in one respect. He had joined a brokerage firm just out of college, and he was so successful as a stock trader that he had become financially secure before his mid-twenties, when his illness forced him to quit working. Now aged 36, he still followed the market closely, though he rarely left his apartment, and his investments yielded a comfortable income. Of course, he was extremely thorough in his investigations of stock issues. After first ferreting out every scrap of information, he agonized over trading decisions. Two rooms in his apartment were full of files and boxes containing back issues of financial publications and annual reports. After an idea for a trade occurred to him, Jerry would immerse himself in study of the company. However, before actually placing his order by calling his broker, he always felt the same old tension increasing. This forced him to check and recheck all his data and calculations. Jerry's indecisiveness did make him miss some opportunities, but his thoroughness more than made up for that.

Jerry never could pinpoint the onset of his illness. When asked, he would say that it had been developing all his life. He had been meticulous as a child, and at different times in his life, certain acts had had to performed with irrational perfection. For example, at age 15 he found that he had to be sure not one drop of urine leaked onto his underwear. He carried cotton swabs to clean himself. The process often took 10 to 15 minutes, and the head of his penis became so tender that he would wince when it brushed his clothing. That preoccupation lasted for several weeks. Months later, he became tormented by a recurring thought: He was going to kill his mother accidentally with a large knife that hung in the kitchen and then dispose of the body by grinding it up, part by part, in the garbage disposal. An introspective boy, Jerry knew that he dearly loved his mother and that the last thing he wanted was to harm her. But the thought came anyhow, tormenting him for hours. He actually pictured his mother dismembered in various ways. He tried to think of other things, but that effort just seemed to make the irresistible thoughts bloodier. This torture went on for nearly a month and then subsided. But the thoughts kept recurring, often in the background of his consciousness for a few seconds, sometimes for a few intense hours. And once or twice a year, they utterly disabled him for days.

By the time Jerry entered college, he was sure something was wrong with him. He had read a lot of psychology books, and had diagnosed himself as having "obsessive-compulsive neurosis" and presented himself to the student health clinic. There followed three years of psychoanalytic psychotherapy, which he thought made him a little better able to cope with the college's academic and social life, but it did not change the basic features of his illness. In fact, things seemed to get worse: Episodes lasted longer, and the recurring thoughts were more intense. He did learn that upsetting events in his life—final examinations, his father's illness—tended to aggravate his condition. He also learned, to his great relief, that he would never actually mutilate his mother or commit similar violent acts that sometimes came unbidden to mind.

While in college, Jerry had his first serious relationships with women. When relatively free of his unnatural thoughts and tension, he was an intelligent and charming companion. Once he nearly became engaged to a popular and active biology major. Their courtship was a conventional one until just before the pair separated for the first weeks of the summer vacation. Jerry went shopping for a present. He had settled on an amount of money he wanted to spend and quickly chose a simple, tasteful bracelet. But before buying it, he was beset by rising tension and indecision. Was the bracelet good enough? Would she like the design? Should he have spent more money? The jeweler let him take three additional bracelets, all more expensive than the original one, on overnight approval. But still unable to choose, that evening Jerry asked his girlfriend to pick one. He showed her all four bracelets, hinting that he preferred his original choice. Perplexed and a little irritated, she chose the most expensive one. Jerry could not hide an involuntary gulp and finally had to explain that the bracelet cost more than he wanted to spend. There followed a major quarrel, but after final exams they made up. She kept the bracelet she had chosen.

Half a year later he decided to propose marriage. He had agonized over the decision, although she had made it clear that she would welcome his proposal. Finally he chose a ring, but again the tension began rising. This time he had the jeweler place the ring on a tray in his display window with four more expensive alternatives, but with Jerry's choice much more prominently displayed. That evening in a park just across from the jeweler, he proposed marriage. With every smile and gesture, she gave unmistakable "yes" signals, but she said she wanted to think about her answer overnight.

The jeweler's shop was closed, but he led her to the window, showed her the rings, and asked her to choose one. Before long, as they looked and discussed the rings, he had to tell her why one ring was set apart from the others. That evening she said little. The next day she told Jerry she never again wanted to see him.

After the three years of psychoanalysis Jerry tried several other treatments, each of which seemed partly effective for a while. These approaches included behavior modification and antidepressant drugs. The drugs did help relieve the depression that sometimes came when he reflected on the life to which his thoughts and cleaning binges condemned him. Sedative drugs, including alcohol, also helped, but not for long. After taking such drugs he became groggy, and he did not like many of the other feelings produced by alcohol.

Diagnosis: Obsessive–Compulsive Disorder

Jerry's self-diagnosis, obsessive-compulsive neurosis, was correct. The modern names for the condition are obsessional illness and obsessive-compulsive disorder. It affects between 1 and 2 percent of the adult population. Jerry's illness was a notably severe one.

Signs and Symptoms

Obsessions

Obsessions are intrusive thoughts or images that are repeated over and over. Like delusions, obsessions are a disorder of thought content. They come unbidden, are usually distressing, and are seen as separate from the usual personality—as "alien," in professional jargon. Jerry's thoughts about dismembering his mother are a fairly typical example. Obsessional thoughts can consume consciousness by blocking out everything else, thus drastically disrupting normal life. Jerry had learned from books and doctors that he would never act on these thoughts. This knowledge helped Jerry, but the thoughts were still terribly distressing.

Compulsions

Compulsions are ritualistic acts, such as Jerry's cleaning binges. An impulse to act comes to mind and must be followed, even though the affected person fully understands that the action commanded is nonsensical. If the command is not followed, anxiety increases to intolerable levels. Affected persons try hard to resist performing compulsive actions and to rid their minds of obsessional thoughts. But any success is temporary. Jerry's illness illustrates the cost of anxiety; his only escape from it was performing his rituals. Neither he nor anyone else understood why he became so irrationally anxious. He knew only that if he did not perform the rituals, his anxiety would become unbearable, whereas if he gave in, he could temporarily escape. He was fully aware of the social and economic costs he had paid and would continue to pay. But he could find no other answer.

Indecision

The indecision illustrated by Jerry's fumbling attempts to buy jewelry for his girlfriend and by the manner of making his stock market transactions, is also a common feature of obsessional illness. Though he knew what he wanted, much of the time Jerry was compelled to agonize over each detail of his reasoning, to review again and again the grounds for the decision. He knew this was an utterly unproductive exercise. But any decision he acted on was followed by intolerable anxiety. Naturally, there had been times when he had successfully forced himself to act quickly, to defy his indecision. He soon gave up such attempts, however, not because rapid action caused mistakes—he had already thought thoroughly about what he wanted to do—but because he suffered such misery afterward. Far from feeling gratified by having overcome his indecision, he agonized, sometimes for days, about the action he had forced himself to take. If the action could be undone, he had to fight, sometimes unsuccessfully, against undoing it.

Of course, obsessions and compulsions in one form or another are features of normal life and ordinary language. Most of us have at some time become anxious because something was dirty and have gone on an unreasonable cleaning spree. Many normal people are scrupulous about cleaning and demand a degree of perfection that seems unreasonable to others. Occasionally at least, most of us are also irrationally indecisive. We even have irrational or bizarre thoughts that flash across our consciousness and then disappear. These thoughts don't persist as Jerry's did, however, and they don't arouse emotion, so most of us don't regard such features of our personalities as the result of illness. They are not dis-ease to us, and we may find it difficult to acknowledge them as disease in others.

Here too, language may encourage lack of empathy with real illness. The way the words *obsession* and *compulsion* are used in everyday speech is only tangentially related to their use as medical diagnostic terms. For example, it is very hard (I think impossible) to include "compulsive gambling" among true compulsions in the medical sense. The aim is financial gain, not relief from anxiety, and the gambling itself is usually experienced as an emotional high, not a miserable chore. Likewise, the phrase "obsessed with love" does not describe an "alien" or irrational feeling. Indeed, being "obsessed" connotes lofty dedication, and being "compulsive" implies that one is very painstaking. Subtle distinctions perhaps, but possibly reasons why this major illness, the cause of so much misery, is so little known and so easily discounted.

Panic, Phobic, and Generalized Anxiety Disorders

These illnesses feature anxiety but not disabling obsessions and compulsions. Variants of each have from time to time been represented in official nomenclatures; agorophobia, social phobia, and simple phobia are current entries. The frequency of all such illnesses combined, in the adult population, has been estimated at 2 to 4 percent; estimates vary widely because the disorders merge into one another and into normal behavior. They usually begin in adolescence or early adult life, though onset in childhood is seen occasionally. After the mid-thirties, the risk for onset becomes low. That is an important diagnostic point. As we have seen, depression can exaggerate what was previously an innocent personality trait until it becomes a major disability that deceptively overshadows the depression itself. Onset of an anxiety disorders after age 30 to 35 suggests that depression or some other brain disease may be the primary disorder and should be sought.

Panic Disorder

Panic disorder affects about one and one-half percent of the adult population. In a panic attack, uncontrollable anxiety begins abruptly. The heart starts pounding, breathing becomes rapid, there is often a sensation of choking or smothering, and the affected person may develop other signs and symptoms of anxiety. Panic attacks would be adaptive in situations that posed real danger, but they do not come at such times. Instead they may come at any time, though they occur more frequently in some situations, such as when an affected person is driving or is in a crowded store. Affected persons realize that there is no real danger and no reason for panic. But attacks cannot be fended off through bravery, or self-trickery, or understanding of their cause. (Remember that anxiety makes a shambles of rational thinking.) The attacks usually last several minutes, but they can go on much longer. They may occur several times daily or they may be quite rare.

The average age at onset of panic disorder is about 25. Females are four times as likely as males to receive this diagnosis, but statistics can mislead. Females may simply be more likely to seek medical help, and males more likely to self-medicate with alcohol.

Panic disorder interferes with normal life, all the more so because the attacks seem so unreasonable to the affected person and those trying to understand him or her. Often a major complication, *anticipatory anxiety*, appears. This means that affected persons begin to dread—and hence to avoid—situations that have given rise to panic. For example, if panic attacks tended to occur when he or she was driving, the victim would come to fear and avoid getting behind the wheel. The result may closely resemble phobic disorder. Hence distinguishing panic disorder from phobic disorder is often hard to do (and probably not helpful). Many ways of subdividing and naming have been proposed and applied, but none has passed the basic test applied to medical diagnoses: None has helped with prognosis or treatment.

Phobia

The term *phobia* denotes intense disabling fear of specific objects or situations. The fear cannot be understood as a reaction to any actual danger; affected people recognize it as irrational, but that does not help them master it. Typical phobias involve spiders, closed spaces, and heights, but nearly any object will serve: cats, water, electricity, safety pins, you name it. If the number of eliciting stimuli is small and relatively discrete, the designation is "simple phobia"—certainly a misleading name. Two other conditions rooted in phobic anxiety are currently classified as subtypes of phobic disorder.

Social Phobia

Social phobia is an irrational fear of such activities as eating in front of others, public speaking, and waiting in lines. Affected people recognize that their fear is groundless, yet they vigorously attempt to avoid situations evoking the fear.

Agoraphobia

This condition is better understood as a complication of some other anxiety disorder than as a separate illness. The term is derived from the Greek *agora*, which means "marketplace." It is applied diagnostically to people who avoid public places and situations—shopping malls, church services, crowds, public transportation. Agoraphobia is due to anticipatory anxiety. For example, if shopping were associated with panic attacks, even the thought of going downtown could cause severe anxiety. Anticipatory anxiety may become an extremely potent motivator, leading affected people to avoid contact with the outside world, thus rendering them virtually housebound. This is agoraphobia.

Generalized Anxiety Disorder

When enough unrealistic anxiety is present to produce dis-ease, while distinguishing features such as phobias or panic episodes are not so prominent as to force a diagnosis of one of the more specific anxiety disorders, the condition is regarded as a generalized anxiety disorder. Generalized anxiety disorder is not usually so disabling as the other anxiety disorders, although affected people are especially prone to worry and are known to friends and relatives as worriers.

Signs and Symptoms

Many of the signs and symptoms marking the anxiety disorders have already been described. However, there are other important manifestations of severe anxiety no matter what its cause. *Depersonalization* is an alteration in perception that makes one's body seem unreal. Often this is experienced as seeing oneself from a distance, as though from a cloud. Sometimes a limb or even one's whole body seems distorted—elongated perhaps, or flattened. In *derealization,* it is objects in the external world that seem distorted. Affected persons are usually greatly distressed by these perceptions. But they know that their perceptions are false, a knowledge that distinguishes depersonalization and derealization from hallucinations. The couch in the corner is not really semiliquid with waves running through it, and the victim knows that he or she is not actually the person seen below as if through the small end of a telescope.

Anxiety can induce too rapid breathing—usually called *hyperventilation* or simply *overbreathing* by professionals. The effect of overbreathing is elimination of too much carbon dioxide, which (as the result of a complex chemistry involving calcium) can produce sensations of tingling and numbness. Often the lips and nearby face are first affected, but fingertips and other skin areas may also be involved. These strange sensations increase anxiety leading to faster breathing and another vicious circle. Breathing into a paper bag is sometimes prescribed as a means of reversing the loss of carbon dioxide. The buildup of carbon dioxide in the bag forces the equilibrium in the opposite direction so that more carbon dioxide is retained in the body. This is often an effective countermeasure, but usually only for a short time. One might think affected persons could voluntarily control their breathing rate and thus reverse the process, but they cannot. I have tried many times to get people to slow their breathing both during an anxiety attack and (as a preventative measure) when an attack threatened. None of my patients has had significant success, probably because anxiety makes it impossible to concentrate on breathing rate.

Prognosis

After onset, the anxiety disorders have a variable course. Most often the disability is tolerably mild, but it may worsen to disabling levels when environmental challenges (a new job, a promotion, unemployment, divorce, school examinations) add further anxiety to a baseline that is already high. This worsening is best seen as the crossing of a threshold; the challenges do not cause the disease, they merely overload an already compromised physiology. For other persons, triggering events cannot be identified: They have a chronic disabling illness that does not change much over time.

Obsessive-compulsive disorder generally begins in adolescence or early adult life. Onset after age 30 to 35 is rare. Once established, it tends to persist for life. However, nearly all cases exhibit distinct swings in severity. Depression worsens obsessive-compulsive disorder, just as it worsens everything else. Generally, people with mild obsessional illness find that they can manage their lives with little disruption and simply pay no attention to what amounts to a personality quirk. Those with even moderately severe obsessional illness, however, often find life difficult and unrewarding. This is partly due to the obsessional thoughts and compulsive behaviors themselves. It is also partly because anyone in close contact with an affected person must tolerate unreasonable intrusions into life's ordinary duties and pleasurable activities. The Jerry's of the world are often alone.

Accumulating evidence from family studies suggests that the anxiety disorders may be components of a disease complex that involves a disturbed balance among several brain neuronal systems wherein serotonin and dopamine are the main neurotransmitters. As noted in Box 3 (page 84), studies of relatives of psychiatric patients have repeatedly turned up several conditions present at rates in excess of those found in the general population. Anxiety disorders, especially obsessional illness, are found in excess among relatives of persons with *Tourette's syndrome*. Tourette's syndrome is characterized by abrupt muscular twitches (called tics) and by explosive, involuntary vocal sounds. It is thought to be associated with over-stimulation of neural networks that use the neurotransmitter dopamine. Several illnesses may be associated with Tourette's syndrome, but just which of these will prove to belong to a defined disease complex is not yet clear. The important point is that the intricate adjustments of brain physiology involved in the anxiety disorders are beginning to become accessible to experimental manipulation—and thus to our understanding. The immediate future looks bright.

Treatment

Although future prospects are good, there are today no specific curative treatments for the anxiety disorders. However, modern techniques of disease management can help most affected persons live normal lives. Mild anxiety disorders can be managed in such a way that they interfere little with ordinary life. Often, making simple adjustments is all that is necessary. For example, an accountant with a severe heights phobia works on the forty-eighth floor of a downtown building. He found that he could not work in an exterior office, but he does perfectly well in an interior one with no windows. Panic attacks can also be avoided. Shopping can be done during hours when there is no crowding, or one can drive on residential streets instead of on freeways. Such practical accommodations to illness may be bothersome, but they are a price well worth paying.

More severe anxiety disorders are generally treated with a combination of psychotherapy and medication. Today, the psychotherapy most often involves one or another form of behavior modification ("behavior mod").

Behavior Modification

There are several different models of behavior modification. One of Jerry's treatments was "implosion therapy," the most radical of those commonly used. The basic procedure is systematic exposure, in carefully graded doses, to whatever stimulus creates dis-ease. In Jerry's case, the exposure was to dirt. The treating psychologist began with a clean dish, which Jerry had to leave on his drainboard. Then dirty items were put on the dish each day—coffee grounds, eggshells, the contents of an ashtray, and so on. Jerry felt increasing anxiety, but with the psychologist and a rather beefy graduate student prepared to restrain him physically, he didn't try to clean. The theory was that as the challenge increased, and with it Jerry's discomfort, a climax of anxiety would eventually be reached. After experiencing that, Jerry would be able to tolerate anything.

After a couple of treatment sessions, Jerry was able to sleep and even to make and eat his breakfast in the kitchen despite the dirty dishes. As a final test, the psychologist brought a urine-stained diaper and wiped the walls and furniture with it. Jerry went wild. He first attempted to flee the apartment, but the door had been bolted. Then he tried to get to his cleaning materials, but they had been taken away. In the end, he spent two days and one night in misery, supervised by the psychologist and graduate students working in shifts. After that, exhausted, he slept. All concerned had worked very hard indeed. They had given the treatment a good try.

Jerry urgently wanted the treatment to work and he was considerably better for about two weeks. But one day a thought recurred over and over, and two days later he was again "compelled" to clean. Over the next days, all of the gains from his treatment evaporated.

Although Jerry's treatment was unsuccessful, behavior modification is often effective in controlling compulsions. In recent years, the basic approach we described has been modified. Successive exposures to the feared objects or situations are more finely graduated, starting with those just tolerable and moving successively toward ever-more-difficult ones. At each step, maladaptive responses are discouraged rather than physically prevented. Sometimes the treatment consists of merely asking the affected person to refrain from the problem behavior. More often, some neutral distraction (such as continuing to play a favorite game) is used. Over time, the staged situations are made more anxiety-provoking.

Similar staged situations are used for phobias. Unhealthy responses—avoidance or flight—are discouraged. Such methods, when applied skillfully so that anxiety is kept within tolerable limits while the intensity of the anxiety-provoking stimuli is increased steadily, have proved reasonably successful. By giving substantial relief from anxiety, these techniques can restore normal or near-normal functioning in everyday life. They are without significant risks and can be repeated as often as needed for years.

Unfortunately, obsessions and panic attacks cannot be treated effectively through behavior modification techniques. Panic attacks usually occur too unpredictably in terms of both time and eliciting circumstances. And obsessions are thoughts, not behavior, so there is no behavior to modify. Considerable work has been done with various forms of "thought stopping," however. For example, an affected person is encouraged to relax completely, often through the use of quasi-hypnotic techniques. Then obsessional thinking is triggered, usually by the therapist who repeats some phrase known to be evocative. After a timed period of free obsessional thinking, the therapist (or a signal such as a bell) commands "STOP!" Immediately, a prearranged pleasurable experience (music, for example) or a positive thought is introduced, which should theoretically be enhanced as the subject achieves a relaxed state. These methods have so far proved ineffective.

Medication

Some 20 to 30 percent of anxiety disorders do not respond to behavioral treatment methods. Then medical treatments are used. If depressed mood is detected, most psychiatrists prescribe antidepressant drugs. If depression is not notable, treatment is based on a sedative, or antianxiety, drug.

The use of one sedative drug, alcohol, extends back into humankind's prehistory. Even into the present century, alcohol, masquerading as medicine, was the effective ingredient in the numberless remedies for anxiety and insomnia sold in drugstores and by traveling salesmen. Today it is used by huge numbers of people to relieve anxiety—and some of them may actually have a diagnosable anxiety disorder. However, alcohol is a poor choice of treatment because it has several undesirable actions. These include, interference with coordination and thinking. The main "advantage" it offers is accessibility.

In the late nineteenth and early twentieth centuries, other drugs began to be used to supplement alcohol. Bromine and, a few decades later, the barbiturates appeared in patent medicines used for sedation. These were effective sedatives, but they had severe toxic side effects and were subject to overuse and consequent addiction. Several decades later in the 1950s, a new class of drugs, the benzodiazepines, was introduced. These drugs proved more effective and less toxic than earlier sedatives, but their addictive potential is at least as great. Today, they are widely used to treat anxiety.

The benzodiazepines include many well-known drugs such as Librium and Valium. They are effective *anxiolytics*—that is, they relieve anxiety. The accompanying table lists the most often prescribed benzodiazepines; today these drugs are by far the most commonly prescribed for anxiety. In America, they are the most widely prescribed of all drugs.

Benzodiazepine drugs can be very effective in the treatment of anxiety disorders. Many affected persons have taken one or another of the benzodiazepines for decades without a hint of toxicity or addiction. But others find that though these drugs induce short periods of relative well-being, the cost is too high. For them, effective doses—doses that relieve anxiety enough to allow full participation in daily life—also produce a mild intoxication. This feeling, while it may be pleasant or even euphoric, is incompatible with performing intellectually demanding social or vocational tasks. In addition, some people develop tolerance to a sedative and find that they must increase the dosage in order to obtain a constant anxiolytic effect. This practice may lead to addiction. For these reasons, most doctors

BENZODIAZEPINE DRUGS

Generic Name	Brand Name	Usual Dose (milligrams)
Aprazolam	Xanax	1–5
Chlordiazepoxide	Librium	15–100
Clorazepate	Tranxene	15–60
Diazepam	Valium	5–30
Lorazepam	Ativan	1–10

prescribe benzodiazepines (or other sedative drugs) for only brief periods, and then only to meet some important treatment objective, such as getting through a period of special stress.

Sedative drugs are somewhat more useful to people with severe phobic disorders than to those with obsessional illness. This is because increases in distress resulting from phobia can be better anticipated. Especially stressful events, such as meetings, journeys, or social ceremonies, can often be foreseen, so a drug can be used as needed to "take the edge off" anxiety. This use of medicine may be frowned on by judgmental persons who view it as providing an unwarranted "crutch." But few such persons have anxiety disorders.

Recently a new medication, *clormipramine*, has been reported to produce great improvement in obsessional illness. The preparation has not yet been approved for use in the United States, but it is available in Canada and Europe. Many Americans who wish to try the drug have found ways to obtain it. So far, the results have been quite encouraging. Most treated cases have reported substantial improvement. (However, there have also been unsuccessful trials, including one by Jerry: He obtained a supply of the drug from Canada and took it for nearly six months before giving up.) Moreover, clormipramine is also an antidepressant, so it is possible that a proportion of those who reported major improvements were people whose primary illness was depression. It takes years to establish that a new drug is both effective and safe. Meanwhile, we suspend judgment but remain hopeful.

Nearly all people with anxiety disorders can manage their problem quite satisfactorily by a treatment regimen combining avoidance of situations difficult for them, commonsense behavior modification, and drugs, both antidepressant and sedative. (Drugs are usually needed only intermittently, but in rare cases, continuous administration is warranted.) However, a small proportion of persons just do not respond to these measures and are left to face decades of illness as incapacitating and distressing as any known. For a selected few of these sufferers, surgery has been helpful.

Psychosurgery

The modern use of surgery for psychiatric disease has its roots in the so-called *frontal lobotomy*. This procedure was developed by a neurosurgeon, Egas Moniz, in the mid-1930s. In 1949 he was awarded a Nobel prize. His operation was first used for intractable illnesses, mainly schizophrenia.

For some patients, surgery suppressed flagrant disorders of thought and reduced anxiety. But for many the price was much too high. The major features of their illness were replaced by a pervasive apathy and neglect of the basics of social deportment. Nevertheless, the procedure became widely used, probably because favorable outcomes were given undue weight in making prognoses. Psychosurgery became available at a time when hospitals were terribly overcrowded and there were no effective treatments other than electroshock. The prognosis without treatment seemed hopeless, and surgery did yield a few favorable outcomes, so why not take the chance? It is estimated that before the mid-1950s, when the procedure fell into disrepute, 40,000 frontal lobotomies were done in the United States. Although the advent of phenothiazine drugs contributed most to its abandonment, few regretted the demise of frontal lobotomy, and for the next couple of decades, psychosurgery effectively ceased in this country.

However, European psychiatrists and neurosurgeons continued to work on a much different surgical approach. They aimed at reproducing frontal lobotomy's positive results without its unacceptable side effects. Toward this end, they devised more refined and discrete operations that made small, precise interruptions in the tracts of nerve tissue that course through the brain establishing communication among cell groups. Some of these tracts were known to be involved with emotion. Gradually, attention focused on the cingulate gyrus, a tract in the frontal midline part of the brain, perhaps a quarter of an inch square in cross section. By the mid-1960s, European centers were reporting encouraging results not with schizophrenia, as had been expected, but rather with the anxiety-related illnesses, including chronic depressions that featured unusually high levels of anxiety. Prodded by these reports, a commission appointed by the National Institutes of Health reintroduced the subject of psychosurgery into the United States. In 1976 the commission's report, endorsed limited investigation into the use of psychosurgery for patients who had not benefited from conventional treatments. This research was to be done only by certain institutions—mainly university hospitals—and was to be supervised by a committee at each institution. The committees were charged with ensuring that the operation was likely to be beneficial, that all conventional treatments had been tried and had failed, that fully informed consent had been obtained, and that careful before-and-after studies were done.

The new surgical procedure, *cingulotomy*, is only distantly related to frontal lobotomy. The surgeon makes a small cut in the cingulate gyrus, using instruments that permit exact localization of the incision within the brain. Two electrodes on the tips of needles are used to make the cut. Minimal openings are made in the skull, and no brain tissue is destroyed except by intent. Exhaustive testing has revealed no loss of memory or of any other intellectual capacity. Epileptic seizures develop in about 10 percent of cases, but these are readily controlled with medications.

The effects of this surgery have been so promising that the procedure is now done routinely at many centers, including the University of Minnesota, where I formerly chaired the Psychosurgery Committee. Like most centers, we found that the procedure produced excellent results (normal functioning) in about 40 percent of the patients who underwent surgery and fair results (some improvement) in 40 percent. The other 20 percent remained unchanged. The best results have been obtained in chronic anxiety with depression (60 percent excellent), the worst with obsessive-compulsive illness (25 percent excellent). It is important to remember that the only people who are candidates for cingulotomy had disabling illness that has failed to respond to all other known treatments. Though it is a treatment of last resort, surgery has earned a small but important—and perhaps permanent—place in psychiatric treatment.

Box 4   Dependence and Invalidism

Beyond certain limits, compassion for and understanding of those suffering from disease can become destructive rather than helpful. Although these limits apply to any illness of any system, the danger of fostering avoidable dependence and invalidism through oversolicitousness is perhaps somewhat greater for the anxiety disorders than for other psychiatric illnesses.

Many illnesses—schizophrenia, rheumatoid arthritis, and multiple sclerosis, for example—tend to worsen over time, and those affected may require constant care and attention. Other conditions—traumatic injuries, stroke, obsessional illness, and manic-depressive illness—do not necessarily worsen because of disease processes themselves. Yet such diseases too often lead to social and economic deterioration, not because of disease directly, but rather because of reactions to it. This may occur no matter what the nature of the original disease or injury and no matter what organ system was affected.

Major illness or injury changes an ill person's whole social milieu as family and friends, and sometimes employers and social agencies, accommodate him or her. Roles change as others take up the responsibilities of the ill person. Some dependence on others is, of course, an inevitable consequence of serious illness. But once established, routines tend to persist, sometimes long after the original humanitarian purpose has been fully served. And the longer dependence continues, the harder it is to reverse. A significant complication that often arises is that both the dependent person and those depended on come to resent their roles.

Professionals sometimes use the demeaning term *secondary gain* to describe such dependence. The "ill" person "gains" attention and nurture from continuing "illness." This pejorative labeling is not constructive. Those who care for the ill person, including health professionals, should rather focus on ensuring that the ill person adapts to the illness in constructive ways and then returns to normal life as rapidly as recovery permits.

Individuals vary widely in their tendency to become dependent. Even after lengthy illness, some rare individuals simply take up life just where it was interrupted, hardly missing a beat. Others have more difficulty and can benefit from professional help with at least two major obstacles. The first of these is deciding what gains to expect and work toward as convalescence proceeds. Often a professional's authoritative estimates are needed. Such an estimate can help families clear the second obstacle too. A working unanimity is needed among family members, the ill person, and all others concerned regarding what can be expected of the recuperating person. Division on this point can be deadly. Communications must be clear. Often convalescent persons who can still achieve great gains in independence truly believe they are as self-sufficient as they can possibly be. They should understand why higher expectations are being set and what those expectations are. So should everyone else concerned. Some caregivers tend to promote dependence and have to restrain themselves. The best way to handle the recovering person's limited capacity to envision beoming more independent is simply to treat it as a normal consequence of illness that betrays no weakness of character.

■ *If You Have an Anxiety Disorder*

When experiencing an anxiety attack, many affected persons feel that they are going to die or lose their minds. The physical distress and disruption of thinking make this fear quite understandable, but remember that those things *will not occur*. Knowing this won't reduce the distress of an actual attack, but many people are beset by such groundless self-doubts when they are between attacks and would otherwise be feeling well. Also be assured that although you will have good and bad months, on average the attacks won't get worse and your condition won't deteriorate. If anything, anxiety disorders tend to improve slowly with time. It is not known whether this gradual improvement reflects an age-related physiologic change or an adaptation to illness. Perhaps it is some of both. You will develop methods that help minimize the effects of anxiety, and you will learn how you can best live with it.

■ *If Someone Close to You Has an Anxiety Disorder*

Always remember that the anxiety underlying these conditions is painful, it is real pain that anyone might experience and it cannot simply be willed away. "Straighten up and fly right" is easy advice to give, but it is unhelpful at best and is sometimes destructive. Affected persons realize that their fears are irrational. They themselves cannot understand their origin, and they certainly don't choose to endure the torture that afflicts them. No one can prevent anxiety from arising; it is an unsummoned physiologic response. We can try to modify how we behave when anxious, and most affected persons try time and again, like Jerry, to ignore the dis-ease they feel so intensely and to behave normally. Any success they may achieve does not last long. Acceptance and tolerance are what they need most, but these must be leavened by common sense. Box 4 describes some of the hazards of over-protection and how to avoid them.

Post-Traumatic Stress Disorder

A new diagnosis that the American Psychiatric Association has recently made official and classified among the anxiety disorders is *post-traumatic stress disorder*, now widely known as PTSD. Any change in diagnostic classification guarantees a flare-up of acrimonious debate in the professional literature. Is the proposed disorder really new? Does it carry with it a useful prognosis? Is it really a disorder or just a variant of the normal? These hard questions have implications extending beyond medicine. Indeed, recent decades have seen the infighting among mental health professionals crowded offstage by claims for compensation championed by clamorous politicians and attorneys. Post-traumatic stress disorder, one of the major enduring legacies of the Vietnam war, continues to spark such battles of its own.

There is no doubt that some signs and symptoms do result from the massive psychological trauma of frontline combat. The salient features of PTSD include intrusive memories, nightmares, flashbacks, and hypervigilance. But is this result abnormal? Wouldn't normal people experience it after such a dose of massive fear in war? Does PTSD differ from the "shell shock" of World War I and the"combat neurosis" of World War II? Why did only a minority of Vietnam veterans develop the disorder? Development of PTSD symptoms is not correlated with degree of exposure to stressful events. Because the environment of wartime combat is so special, doing the systematic research needed to answer such questions well enough to refine and establish a diagnostic entity is not practical. However, for good or ill, the problem has been taken up by civilian medicine.

Among civilians, the trauma leading to PTSD must be, according to the American Psychiatric Association, "an event outside ordinary human experience that would be markedly distressing to almost anyone." Several examples are named; they include rape, physical assault, and seeing someone killed. However, these presumed predisposing events are very widespread within the population: About 40 percent of all adults have experienced one or more of them. Of that 40 percent, 25 percent describe enough symptoms to warrant a diagnosis of PTSD. This means that 10 percent (25 percent of 40 percent) of the total adult population have PTSD. It also means that 75 percent of those at risk because they experienced major trauma do not develop PTSD. For those who do develop PTSD, the symptoms tend to recede over time. The 25 percent holds for the first month, but by one year after the traumatic event, 12 percent, almost half of those affected, are free or nearly free of symptoms. Rape is the traumatic event by far the most predictive of PTSD, and it is the one associated with the most persistent dis-ease. About 80 percent of all women who are raped develop PTSD.

Little is known about the effects of traumatic events other than rape, except that they are far weaker predictors of PTSD. It is known that there is no increase in other diagnoses among those with PTSD. It has been claimed that rates of alcoholism, drug abuse, and depression increase among those affected by PTSD, but the base rates of those problems in the general population are so high that sheer coincidence easily explains why some persons exhibit both PTSD and one of those other disorders. Finally, among civilians, as among those who have survived military combat, there appears to be a susceptible subgroup: People who develop PTSD after trauma tend to have an excess of pre-existing anxiety disorders over people who do not develop PTSD.

Obviously, scientific knowledge of PTSD is unsatisfying, and untangling the medical condition from the web of politics that surrounds compensation for war injury—and increasingly for civilian injury—will take research and time. Even in so-called hard sciences, progress must sometimes wait until passions have cooled. At present, no effective treatment for PTSD is known, but some authorities think that counseling helps make the dis-ease more bearable.

4

DRUG ABUSE

∎∎∎

From the settlements of ancient Mesopotamia to Park Avenue penthouses, our species has demonstrated unquenchable resolve to alter brain function by any available method. We have rewarded with immense fortunes those who supply us with alcohol, nicotine, caffeine, cocaine, and other "mind-bending" substances that are well known, at least by name, to nearly everyone over the age of six. But water is used for this purpose too. Drink enough of it over a short enough period of time and you get a "buzz." Some of us actually keep ourselves intoxicated with water. Aspirin, which produces a "glow," is fairly commonly used for non-medical purposes. So are many other inexpensive drugs with innocent reputations. Reducing the brain's supply of oxygen by choking off its blood supply is practiced in an effort to produce a sexual "high." (Accidental death by hanging is one occasional side effect.) Because the quickest and easiest route to the brain is through the lungs, inhaling drugs is especially popular. Gasoline fumes are used by ghetto youths, anesthetic gases by affluent medical personnel. Inhalation of vaporized cocaine, "crack," by all social classes threatens our civil order.

The term commonly employed to describe the use of drugs in ways or in amounts that are not socially sanctioned is *drug abuse*. *Non-medical,* or *recreational, use* are equivalent terms. Just how abuse is defined depends in large part on social factors. This is inconvenient for those who seek absolute definitions, but it is true nevertheless. For example, the argument for banning tobacco is at least as strong as the case for banning any other addicting drug. Tobacco damages health. Because it causes fires and environmental contamination, it is dangerous to nonsmokers. Tobacco is highly addicting; many smokers have as little effective control over their use of their drug as any heroin addict. Promotion of tobacco by advertisements and free samples distributed by personable young men and women has been at least as effective as the methods used by the legendary "pushers" of heroin. Yet despite the evidence, tobacco was (until recently) accepted in nearly all social circles. Users expected to be free to smoke at any time and to have matches and ashtrays available everywhere.

Suddenly, in the industrial West, attitudes are being transformed. Virtually overnight, tobacco use has been widely acknowledged as drug abuse and dis-ease. Yet at the same time, in much of the non-Western world, a change in the opposite direction is taking place: Use of tobacco is increasing, and smoking is considered neither drug abuse nor dis-ease.

History provides many other examples of changing definitions of drug abuse. Drinking alcohol was once forbidden by law in the United States and is today illegal in most Muslim countries. During certain periods in America and Europe, cocaine, heroin, and amphetamine were widely used as legal or quasi-legal drugs. Changes and inconsistencies in social perspective pepper the history of the human species' relationship to drugs.

Tolerance, dependence, withdrawal, and *addiction*—these terms are critical to understanding abuse of nearly all the drugs we will be discussing, yet they are not well understood by the public or by many professionals.

Tolerance to a drug means that after repeated administration, a given dose of that drug no longer produces the same effect. Or, put another way, dosage must be increased in order to produce a constant effect. Tolerance depends on three mechanisms: (1) The body's ability to eliminate the drug is increased, mainly because the liver increases its production of chemicals that destroy the drug. Thus more drug is needed to overcome this enhanced efficiency. (2) The physiologic system affected by the drug acts to neutralize its effects. Legend tells us that medieval poisoners took, over time, increasing doses of their favorite poisons in order to become able to tolerate doses fatal to their victims. They could then share a last meal without arousing suspicion. (3) Behavioral mechanisms develop that tend to neutralize the effects of the drug taken. For example, narcotics depress respiration. In response, unconscious reflex mechanisms act to increase the breathing rate of an experienced user just before a narcotic is injected. The body prepares. These behavioral mechanisms depend on environmental stimuli that alert the body to expect a drug. This aspect of tolerance can kill. It is likely that many deaths resulting from injection of narcotics—heroin especially—are not due to overdoses. Rather, the dose is one previously tolerated by the user, but because of some change in environmental signals—perhaps just using the drug in unfamiliar surroundings—the body is not adequately prepared. Sudden death results.

It is most important to note that drugs have multiple effects and that tolerance to each effect may develop separately to different degrees, and at different rates in different persons. For example, stimulant drugs commonly elevate mood and suppress appetite. Tolerance to these two effects develops separately and at different rates: for one person, rapidly for mood elevation, slower for appetite suppression; for another person, the opposite. The outcome is that a whole series of adaptations to several effects of drugs occurs before and after drug administration, and these vary from person to person.

Dependence is the condition exhibited by a user who has undergone some combination of the physiologic and behavioral changes we have noted that compensate for the effects of a drug. If no drug or too little drug is administered, these compensatory changes produce discomfort or even severe illness. This is known as *withdrawal*. The signs and symptoms of withdrawal vary from drug to drug. Moreover, a drug-dependent person is not only controlled physically by the drug (because of withdrawal) but is also controlled psychologically and socially. Obtaining drugs in order to both experience desired effects and avoid withdrawal becomes a central activity in life. Drugs that are abused tend to be *reinforcing*. That is, animals—including man—when tested under strict laboratory conditions, will do work in order to obtain the drug. (In contrast, animals will not work for major tranquilizers or most antidepressants; they will instead work to avoid them. These are unpleasant drugs to take.)

Addiction is a controversial term that today has little scientific utility. As used by the World Health Organization, it is defined as the use of drugs to avoid withdrawal. Thus an addict is one who is dependent on a drug. This definition is uncomfortably circular, but *addiction* serves well enough as popular shorthand for the complex biologic relationships described above.

Many drugs share characteristics that permit us to group them together as a class. Drugs belonging to the same class share similar properties, among the most useful of which is that they can be substituted for one another. This means that withdrawal from one drug can be prevented by use of another drug in the class; alcohol withdrawal is often treated with Valium or a similar drug. A further implication is that the effects of drugs in the same class are additive; for example, using alcohol and Valium together increases one's intoxication. This section begins with a chapter on alcohol and other drugs classed as sedatives. The following chapter describes stimulant, hallucinogenic, and narcotic drugs.

Alcohol, by far the most widely used sedative, is ubiquitous in our society. We drink to "drown our sorrows," but also to celebrate. We use it to relax but also to put us into a party mood. As a drug, alcohol is actually a depressant—in fact, it is an anesthetic. It depresses higher brain functions, freeing us somewhat from inhibitions.

Chapter

6

Abuse of Alcohol and Other Sedatives

□ □ □

❏ *Julia*

As far back as she could remember, alcohol was a major factor in Julia's life. Both of her parents drank six or eight cocktails or bottles of beer nearly every evening. After a couple of hours of drinking, they often had loud arguments. Sometimes these escalated into physical battles. Julia, an only child, managed to adapt reasonably well. She was a bright, attractive girl who was eager to please, sensitive to criticism, and always self-sufficient beyond her years. She did well in school and had many friends. Until she was 14 years old, she thought her home was fairly normal.

One Saturday night her parents were in an automobile collision. Her mother was killed and her father's brain was so severely injured that he spent the remaining 15 years of his life in a nursing home. A couple in the other automobile was also killed. Blood samples from all four persons were found to contain high levels of alcohol. Which automobile caused the accident was never established.

Julia went to live with her father's brother. He was 11 years younger than her father, so his two children were much younger than Julia. Julia became more of a live-in baby sitter than she would have liked, but she also felt secure and knew she was making a contribution to the family. Her uncle had been an adamant teetotaler since his adolescence because, he said, he had seen enough tragedy caused by alcohol. He told Julia that he had learned early in life that he could never drink.

In high school Julia became an unusually responsible student-citizen, active in student government, a volunteer librarian, and a good student. A personable girl, she had several friends, including some of the more serious and studious boys. But she parried all requests for dates and rejected any suggestions that she participate in parties. "Prim" was a word used to describe her. Finally, when she was nearly age 17, she began to accept invitations to movies and dances.

One night she went to a party and, for the first time, drank alcohol. Although at first she disliked the taste of the wine that was served, she soon began to feel exhilarated and unrestrained in a way she never had before. She continued to drink, eventually right out of a wine bottle. Relaxed and happy, she seemed to experience hours of hilarious fun. Fortunately, she had arranged to stay that night with a girlfriend, who managed to get her home and into bed. Julia stayed awake happily talking until her hostess fell asleep. Then Julia, who knew the house well, went to a bar in the recreation room and poured a glass of vodka, which she took to bed with her. Finally, after drinking most of the vodka in her glass, she fell asleep.

The next morning, as she reconstructed the events of the night before, she realized that her reaction to alcohol was much different from that of her friends. Her memories of her parents, the hints her uncle had dropped, the reading she had done, and her own new experience combined to make it clear that for her, alcohol was a special hazard. She vowed never to drink again.

The next ten years were busy ones. Julia went through nursing school and became a registered nurse. During her last year in school, she met and married a hospital administrator. For the next six years she successfully combined marriage and career; her marriage was increasingly happy, and she rose to a supervisory position in the surgical operating room. Meanwhile, her husband's career also flourished. When he was named president of a medium-sized hospital, they agreed they wanted to start a family. She stopped working and had two children within two years.

There then began what Julia would later call her nightmare years. She wasn't quite sure how they started. Maybe she never really recovered from her second pregnancy, or maybe it was giving up her job, and the status that accompanied it, in order to be at home with her children. Whatever the reason, she felt increasingly dissatisfied with her life. Even so, she tried with all the energy and skill she could muster to be the perfect mother and wife. Her husband's position required that she be socially active—attend parties, entertain, join volunteer groups, and help in the hospital's fund-raising drives. She felt increasingly ill at ease and socially inept, which was especially hard to bear because she loved her husband and desperately wanted him to succeed in his career.

Of course, alcohol was everywhere. Julia had learned to pretend to drink while actually taking only tiny sips of wine or a half-glass of champagne on ceremonial occasions. At parties she managed to drink only orange juice or ginger ale. Fortunately, her husband was also a light drinker. She disliked what she saw alcohol doing to others, but at the same time she was envious of the relaxed fun they seemed to enjoy. Imperceptibly, her sips of wine increased.

One day when her husband was away in another city, Julia was scheduled to entertain at a luncheon for the volunteers who operated the hospital's gift shop. These volunteers were older women, many born to wealth, all well off and socially important. Julia dreaded the occasion. Although she knew how to entertain, somehow she couldn't relax. Just before the luncheon, she drank half a glass of whiskey and ate a handful of mints. The luncheon went very well. Julia knew she had been charming and loquacious. She had had a glass of wine during the lunch, and she had several more after her guests had left, because she felt that she deserved congratulations.

The luncheon marked a major change in Julia. She became convinced that she could control her drinking after all. Relief from social tension was at hand, so why suffer? Over the next few weeks, she began having a drink or two or three most evenings, and sometimes she drank during the day. She used vodka mixed with orange juice so the drinking would not be obvious, and for a time it was not. Indeed, she seemed much more relaxed to her friends and especially to her husband. He soon learned that she had increased her drinking—though not the true extent of the increase. Thinking it harmless, he began to join her in evening cocktails, which became a ritual of their daily life.

This pattern appeared to continue unchanged for more than a year, but in fact Julia's drinking pattern was changing insidiously. She began increasing her afternoon and evening drinking. To facilitate this habit, she sought out women with whom to have lunch preceded by a martini or two.

The next summer Julia had a lot of free time. She hired a high school girl to watch the children, freeing herself to spend most afternoons sipping wine with friends at a swimming pool. At home she became more irritable, particularly with her husband and especially when he began to question her drinking. "You're always away," she would tell him. "All my friends like a social drink, so if I'm going to have company, I have to join them. Besides, who are you to control me? You drink just as much as I do!" One night she passed out and spent the night sleeping in her garden. A week later she became obviously drunk at a party, spilled a glass of red wine on her hostess's cream sofa, and fell down a half-flight of stairs. The next day she could remember arriving at the party, but everything else was a blur or was missing entirely.

Julia's slide continued. She started every day with wine and finished with several highballs of whiskey or vodka. Later she estimated her intake at one quart of whiskey, or the equivalent, per day. She was hardly involved anymore with the management of her home and family. There were other embarrassing public scenes. Her husband, her friends, and her uncle tried to help her stop drinking, but Julia reacted angrily to these attempts. Her husband took the children to stay with his parents.

There were times when she did attempt to control her drinking, usually by just cutting down the amount, but twice she tried to quit entirely. She found that she could not manage either method. She could not cut down, because when she started drinking, she couldn't stop until she was drunk. And she could not stop entirely, because when she tried, she became intolerably anxious or depressed, or both.

One day, following an afternoon of drinking, she went out in her automobile to pick up some cleaning. On her way she scraped a parked car and then careened into an intersection where she collided with a moving van. She sustained a broken leg, rib and lung injuries, and lacerations. She was taken to a hospital and was later charged with drunken driving.

Julia's injuries were not life-threatening, but she needed an operation to set her broken leg, and the lung injuries required close observation. By the third day in the hospital Julia was feeling reasonably well. However, that evening she began to feel apprehensive and agitated: she spent the night tossing about, sleeping little. By morning she was weak, tremulous, and so nauseated that she was unable to eat or drink. During the day she began to have horrible nightmares, which continued even when she thought she was fully awake. Horrible "string-like tentacles" threatened to envelop her. Noises in the hallway seemed to be sounds of a great battle. Huge, ugly bugs crawled about on her. Her physicians treated her for delirium tremens (DTs), a major consequence of alcohol withdrawal. After another two days, about which Julia mercifully would have only hazy memories, she fell asleep. Two days later she awakened extremely weak but otherwise well. Without question or objection, she accepted transfer to a chemical dependence treatment unit. The same day she received a divorce petition from her husband.

Julia became a model chemical dependence patient. She was ready to acknowledge that alcohol had destroyed the life she had built and that she suffered from a disease—that she was forever an alcoholic. She accepted that she could never again drink alcohol. Even the divorce seemed fitting, though sad. The marriage had suffered so much that she really did not think she could resume it. Her children, who visited regularly and even participated in some of the treatment meetings, seemed truly to appreciate her effort to overcome what they too saw as a sickness. They would live with their father for the immediate future but would visit often. Julia shuddered when she realized how close she had come to losing them too. After a month of treatment, Julia was ready to leave. She joined a chapter of Alcoholics Anonymous (AA).

Julia completed a program to reinstate her nursing license and accepted a position as a general-duty nurse in a clinic. She liked her job but found it stressful. The clinic was busy, and she was given a lot of responsibility for some difficult procedures. She managed well, but at the price of becoming somewhat overly meticulous. Though she always seemed composed, unanticipated problems, which seemed never to cease coming, caused her to be anxious much of the time. She began to review her workday at night in bed and to have trouble getting to sleep.

One Friday afternoon a patient had a seizure while Julia was removing sutures from a surgical wound. She was in no way to blame for this, but she was alone in the clinic, and the past week had been especially hard. Distraught, frustrated, and agitated, Julia somehow took care of her patient and then began to sob uncontrollably. Without really thinking, she walked over to a large bin that the clinic personnel used as a receptacle for drug samples from pharmaceutical companies. She removed half a dozen packages of Valium and immediately took two 5-milligram tablets.

Relief from tension came quickly, and Julia went to her apartment feeling snugly warm, relaxed, and pleasantly giggly. The next evening before a party she took another two tablets, and during the next week, she downed the rest. She recognized the danger but, as before, argued with herself that it was silly to deny herself relief from the pain she felt. However, she had learned a great deal. At the next AA meeting, she stood up and confessed to the membership.

Julia never again took alcohol or any other sedative drug. The years went by, her children grew up, and she eventually developed a highly satisfying long-term relationship with another hospital administrator who happened to be a member of her AA group. After a hectic time at the clinic, she may glance at the bin containing the drugs or at a vial of injectable narcotic. At these times she aches with longing. But she has not slipped.

Diagnosis: Alcoholism

Julia was an addicted alcoholic. Alcohol dependence would be the official diagnosis in her case. This term is too limited, however, because many people who have major problems with alcohol are not dependent—they do not suffer withdrawal when deprived of alcohol. Alcohol abuse is the official diagnosis applicable to such cases, but it is hard to define. Many attempts to establish criteria for the diagnosis of alcohol abuse have been made but none has proved satisfactory. Sheer intake of alcohol fails on one main count: A prognosis based on intake is too inaccurate to be useful because the effects of a given dose of alcohol are too variable from person to person and even in the same person at different times. At one extreme, to those like Julia, use of any alcohol at all is dis-ease. AA's entire treatment philosophy is based on this view. However, that diagnostic standard would apply to only a minority of adults who drink. An overwhelming proportion of adults in the industrial West drink, but most do not feel distress because of it. They feel no dis-ease. Some drink heavily for decades without demonstrable ill effect. What, then, do we use as diagnostic criteria? Two other basic approaches have been developed.

Alcohol and Behavior

This approach focuses on the behavioral consequences of drinking, such as absence from work, the sneaking of drinks, impaired work performance, arguments, violent behavior, and (especially) drunken driving. Arrests for drunken driving bring drinkers into the legal system, and this has led to demands for objective definitions of behavioral impairment related to drinking. Blood alcohol levels have become the objective measurement; the accompanying table describes behaviors associated with various levels of alcohol in the blood.

Enforcement of the law requires specific numbers, but in practice things are not so simple. The level of alcohol in the blood is not a perfect indicator of the amount ingested or of its behavioral effects. The rate of absorption of alcohol from the digestive system depends on many factors, especially the amount and type of food eaten. Food slows absorption. In most social situations, the rapidity with which

BLOOD ALCOHOL LEVELS RELATED TO BEHAVIOR

Blood Alcohol Level[1]	Degree of Intoxication	Notes
0–50	Not intoxicated	3 oz of whiskey/150-lb man
50–200	Mild to moderate (slurred speech)	150 is often the limit for driving[2]
201–300	Obviously drunk (muscle incoordination)	
301–400	Very severe	Often unconscious
over 400	May be fatal	At 800, death highly likely

[1]In milligrams of alcohol per 100 cubic centimeters of blood.
[2]For most legal purposes, the blood alcohol level is determined from expired air. The level of alcohol in expired air is 0.05% of the blood level.

alcohol is ingested affects blood level more than the total amount ingested; the faster the ingestion, the higher the level. And finally, the same blood alcohol level affects behavior differently depending on whether that level is rising or falling. Intoxication is greater when it is rising.

Alcohol Addiction

The second approach to the definition of alcoholism is based on addiction, or, more accurately, on dependence. An individual's progress toward undisputed addictive alcoholism happens in four roughly definable stages, each of which may last from weeks to years.

- *Stage 1* features relief from inner tension. This leads to increasing frequency of drinking and to pleasurable anticipation of drinking as a way to relax.

- *Stage 2* is characterized by daily, often surreptitious intake of alcohol. Avid drinking—gulping a drink or two—is common.

Alcoholic "blackouts," the loss of memory, or hazy memory only, of events that occurred while one was drinking—usually are first seen during this stage.

• *Stage 3* is mainly defined by secret drinking and loss of control of drinking; once begun, drinking cannot be stopped short of drunkenness or exhaustion of supply. The affected person is frequently drunk in the evenings and on weekends, and relationships with family, friends, and co-workers deteriorate.

• *Stage 4* is defined by withdrawal phenomena, especially morning drinking. The accompanying table lists the major features of withdrawal that are observable in alcoholics after a spree of heavy drinking.

In long-standing severe alcoholism, withdrawal syndromes worsen. Seizures (rum fits) may occur. So may a paranoid state with features like those described in Chapter 3. Julia had the most serious withdrawal syndrome of all, delirium tremens (DTs), which may include vivid and terrifying hallucinations (especially visual ones), extreme agitation, and disorientation. Before modern treatment was available, delirium tremens often ended in death; it is still a medical

THE MORNING AFTER:
THE MAJOR FEATURES OF ALCOHOL WITHDRAWAL

Sign or Symptom	Percent of Alcoholics Exhibiting It (grouped by intensity of signs or symptoms)		
	Disabling	Moderate	Mild
Hangovers	84	12	4
Nervousness	83	14	3
Nausea or vomiting, or both	74	19	6
Irritability	70	20	10
Hypersensitivity to noise	62	24	14
Tremors	60	21	19
Drinking to avoid withdrawal	43	36	21

emergency. The condition develops two to three days after drinking is stopped. Julia's experience when she was admitted to the hospital after her accident was typical. In such circumstances doctors may not suspect the extent of the victim's dependence on alcohol, so withdrawal, which could easily be prevented, goes on to full-blown DTs.

In the United States, one or the other of the two official diagnoses, alcohol dependence and alcohol abuse, has been found applicable to 7 to 8 percent of the adult population. Males are about six times as likely as females to receive such a diagnosis. Alcoholism also inflicts immense burdens—financial, social, medical—that thousands of families know all too well. Alcohol addiction and alcohol abuse are two of the world's most important diseases.

"Secondary" Alcoholism

We have seen how people with other illnesses, especially depression or mania, may drink heavily in an apparent effort to self-medicate: a phenomenon known as "secondary alcoholism." This pattern of drinking can closely resemble primary alcoholism, so once again, accurate diagnosis depends on determining which came first, alcoholism or another disorder that led to alcoholism. And again, age at onset is an important clue. Problem drinking typically begins in adolescence or early adult life. If it begins in the fifth decade of life or later, another disease predisposing to excessive use of alcohol may well be present. Successful treatment of that disease usually results in the disappearance of problem drinking. So it was with John, as we saw in Chapter 1. But a primary illness that causes problem drinking cannot usually be recognized until alcohol is completely withdrawn.

Many alcoholics complain of depressed mood, and a few do exhibit signs or symptoms that strongly suggest major depression. But most often depression in alcoholics is an understandable result of what alcohol has done to their lives. And although there are notable exceptions, most problem drinkers have only a single psychiatric problem, alcoholism, from which many other problems result.

Alcohol and Health

Alcohol directly affects every tissue in the body, producing complications in most of them. The organs most severely affected seem to vary somewhat from person to person. The brains of some people are especially vulnerable; in others, it is the liver or pancreas or the peripheral nerves. But there are many complicating factors. For example, alcohol is often combined with other drugs. Nearly all alcoholics are heavy smokers, and many are regular users of recreational drugs other than alcohol. The indirect effects of alcoholism also lead to serious disease. Alcoholics may get the bulk of their calories from alcohol and become vitamin- and protein-deficient. This can lead to severe brain diseases: *Wernicke's disease*, which is a result of thiamine deficiency, and *Korsakoff's disease*, which is probably also due to malnutrition. Alcohol, with its associated malnutrition, is well known as a cause of cirrhosis of the liver, a major disease that destroys the architecture of the liver, compromising the normal passage of blood and bile through it. Indeed, in many studies, the frequency of deaths due to cirrhosis of the liver has been used as an indirect indicator of the frequency of severe alcoholism. Alcohol is not the only cause of cirrhosis, but it far exceeds all others combined.

Alcohol certainly affects the developing unborn children of mothers who drink. During pregnancy, as little as 30 ml (1 oz) of alcohol a day can result in decreased birth weight, and even moderate drinking can lead to an increased rate of spontaneous abortion. In the United States, one or two babies per thousand live births are affected by *fetal alcohol syndrome*. These children are small at birth and remain small for their age. They are mentally handicapped—their average IQ is 63 compared to 100 for the general population—and they are marked by a characteristic facial expression, probably because in their mother's womb, alcohol interfered with the development of their facial bones.

Treatment

No treatment has been effective for alcoholism except abstinence. The basic premise of AA is that alcoholics have a biologic vulnerability to alcohol, that their metabolic systems are different from those of other people, and that therefore they cannot drink. No better answer has been found. Moreover, like Julia, most alcoholics are vulnerable to other sedative drugs and often to narcotics as well.

One drug, disulfiram (Antabuse) has secured a limited place in treatment. Taken daily, this drug produces severe gastrointestinal upset if alcohol is subsequently ingested, and this makes drinking most unpleasant. The drug's effect persists for a couple of days, so it is generally not feasible to omit a morning dose in order to drink that night. Antabuse sounds like an ideal answer, but it has never lived up to its promise. I have found that alcoholics who are able to abstain do so without Antabuse and that those who are not able to abstain discontinue the drug and then drink despite any discomfort. Antabuse may be more effective for the "spree drinker." Such drinkers often begin a drinking bout on impulse. Antabuse may protect them, because knowing that the drug is present in their bodies may make them think again before taking that fateful first drink.

In the past, medical organizations and AA have had public and emotional disagreements about how best to treat alcoholism. Doctors emphasized medical treatments, whereas AA relied on group and family support coupled with intense distrust of drugs that act on the brain. Recently, much better understanding between the two sides has been developing. Doctors acknowledge that they have not developed an effective medical treatment for alcoholism, and most AA chapters now realize that some alcoholics have other illnesses that need drug treatment. All agree that successful treatment usually requires first withdrawing alcohol completely and then treating any other illness present.

AA began as a rigid organization that many alcoholics found incompatible with their convictions or personal styles. This has been changing, however, and anyone who wants to make a sincere effort to defeat chemical dependence can find an AA group suited to his or her needs.

Other Sedative Drugs

Alcohol, barbiturates, and anxiolytic (antianxiety) drugs such as Valium are classified as sedatives. They are among the most often prescribed and most heavily used of all drugs. Surveys have revealed that in America, 11 to 13 percent of adults have taken sedative drugs other than alcohol during the preceding year and that about 2.5 percent take them constantly—every day or nearly every day. The same surveys found, however, that nearly all of the prescriptions written for sedative drugs are medically appropriate. Thus these extremely useful drugs are most often used wisely. But unwise use can lead to serious problems.

Tolerance and Withdrawal

Sedative drugs are reinforcing, and they induce tolerance in many persons who use them. Tolerance to the antianxiety effect or the euphoric effect, or both, then leads to taking increasing doses, until eventually intoxicating doses are attained. Intoxication with all sedative drugs produces much the same result as alcohol: slurred speech, poor coordination, impaired mental functions. No longer taking the drug or reducing the dosage leads to signs and symptoms of withdrawal similar to those associated with alcohol: increasing anxiety, agitation, irritability, nausea, vomiting, weakness, tremors, rapid pulse, increasing blood pressure, convulsive seizures, delirium, and sometimes death. The sedative drugs are the only group of abused substances that carry a risk of death because of the direct effects of withdrawal.

Many pathways lead to abuse of sedative drugs. A frequent one is this: A sedative prescribed for sleep works well at first, but soon the dose is increased because of tolerance. Then a pill or two is taken in the morning to relieve anxiety. This process goes on until very large doses are readily tolerated. If the dose is reduced, anxiety and sleeplessness result. This distress is probably due to withdrawal, but it may be so similar to the dis-ease that led to prescription of the drug in the first place that it can deceive patients and doctors into thinking that the original problem is re-emerging and that increased dosage is needed—a dangerous trap that can insidiously lead to chronic abuse. Eventually, if dosage is increased enough, intoxication results. People vary greatly in their ability to tolerate sedative drugs without exhibiting signs of intoxication. But for everyone, there is a threshold that is eventually crossed if dosage is continuously increased. And there is another important trap for the unwary. If taking the drug is stopped after intoxication appears, the addicted person usually feels well for the first day or two as the drug is cleared from the body. Then, just as the addicted person is indulging in self-congratulation, withdrawal sets in.

Treatment

Withdrawal from sedative drugs is life-threatening and requires expert medical attention. In general, an equivalent dose of another sedative drug is substituted for the problematic drug. This approach is used because the psychological effects of the substituted drug are usually detectably different from those of the original drug and are not so reinforcing to the patient. The dose of the substitute drug is reduced at a standard rate, often 10 percent per day. Withdrawal accomplished in this way is uncomfortable but safe. However, the fact that drug abusers often take a medley of drugs of different classes complicates the management of withdrawal.

In the next chapter we will consider other abused drugs and what we as individuals can do about the huge problems that drugs pose in our society.

7

Abuse of Stimulant, Hallucinogenic, and Narcotic Drugs

□ □ □

THE NON-MEDICAL use of the drugs described in this chapter—stimulants, hallucinogens, and narcotics—is epidemic. In 1988, 14.5 million Americans acknowledged using one or more "street" drugs of these classes during the preceding 30 days. Coping with the effects of these drugs is an enormous drain on the medical system; in 1989, 67,145 emergency room visits were attributable to cocaine or heroin alone. Drug offenses are close to overwhelming the criminal justice system. In 1989, there were 999,381 arrests for drug-related crimes. Of persons arrested for felonies in our large cities, an average of 40 percent test positive for cocaine, 30 percent for amphetamine, and 10 percent for narcotics. These drugs are involved in 73 percent of burglaries, 75 percent of robberies, and 56 percent of assaults and homicides. And beyond the reach of these statistics are social and human costs that cannot be calculated.

Stimulant Drugs

Among the drugs classified as stimulants, only two—cocaine and amphetamine—pose significant psychiatric risks. A third stimulant, caffeine, may produce increased anxiety in susceptible individuals, but cocaine and amphetamine affect all who are exposed to them, sometimes disastrously. Stimulants produce multiple effects. They heighten alertness, decrease fatigue, and elevate mood, sometimes to euphoric levels. They also increase the user's spontaneity, initiative, confidence, and sense of well-being. The stimulants are extremely powerful reinforcers. Animals will literally work themselves to death to obtain more drug. In addition, athletic performance is improved, appetite is suppressed, sexual arousal is enhanced, and apparent need for sleep is reduced. Unwanted toxic effects are usually manifested as a hyperexcited, intense, paranoid state that sometimes closely resembles acute schizophrenia.

Cocaine and amphetamine have the same net effect behaviorally and pharmacologically, but they exert that effect by slightly different mechanisms. Amphetamine increases release of the neurotransmitters dopamine and norepinephrine from vesicles in nerve cells, thereby stimulating the postsynaptic neurons. Cocaine prevents the reuptake of the same two neurotransmitters and that of an additional one, serotonin. It is thought that cocaine's main effect is to block autoreceptors (see Figure 1). This prevents transmitting neurons from obtaining information about the concentration in the synaptic cleft of the neurotranmitter that they release, so they continue to release neurotransmitter. (In technical terms, feedback inhibition is impaired.) Thus, the effects of those three neurotransmitters in the brain are increased. For both amphetamine and cocaine, the excess dopamine they provide to receiving neurons is thought to be by far the most important inducer of euphoria.

The intensity of the effect of stimulant drugs is proportional to the rate at which their concentration increases in the brain, and the most rapid increase is produced via inhalation. Inhaled drug goes from the lungs directly to blood that is bound for the brain. All other means of access to circulating blood that are available to recreational users are slower. Injected drug goes through veins, which return blood to the heart. From there it is pumped into the lungs, back to the heart, and then finally to the brain as one of the destinations of the heart's output. This longer journey means greater opportunity for chemical detoxification and greater dilution. The result is that in the United States, smoking has become a preferred route of administration for cocaine. "Freebasing"—smoking cocaine—produces an onset of action within about 10 seconds and yields very rapid increases in brain concentration. "Crack," a mix of cocaine with baking soda and water, is much simpler to prepare and administer than free base and has largely replaced it. The mixture reduces burning temperature, making inhalation more efficient and comfortable. In some localities crack is being challenged by "crank" or "ice," both of which are inhaled amphetamine. This is an ominous development. Although cocaine is readily available, it does have to be imported, so obtaining a supply subjects users to some risk, however small. Amphetamine can be made in any kitchen.

Although intravenous injection and sniffing (snorting) of cocaine produce a slower rise in the brain's concentration of drug, these methods are still popular with some users. Snorting is the simplest route of administration, mainly because the drug can be used any time and almost anywhere with no special preparation. Snorting is hard on the nose, because the drug constricts blood vessels, shutting off oxygen, and this can lead to destruction of the nasal septum. Intravenous injection is used mainly by older addicts who have become accustomed to injecting themselves; younger users tend to dislike needles. There is additional risk when stimulants are taken by injection, because they produce a sharp rise in blood pressure. Pain due to failure of circulation of blood to the heart is fairly common, as is fatal stroke or heart attack.

Oral ingestion has the slowest onset of action—about 30 minutes. That is why South American Indians can chew coca leaves all day long, obtaining a large daily dose of cocaine but experiencing only mild stimulation (roughly equivalent to that of coffee drinkers).

History yields important perspectives on the current stimulant abuse epidemic. America has been through it all before, including the use of inhaled cocaine. Cocaine was freely available from about 1865, when the active drug was purified in Europe, until 1914, when the Harrison Anti-Narcotic Act became law. It was sold in drugstores as inhalants of relatively pure drug and in "coca cheroots," which were smoked. It was the main flavoring ingredient and stimulant in several patent medicines and in Coca Cola. (In 1905, cocaine was replaced by caffeine in "Coke.") Through this period, medical authorities, including Sigmund Freud, extolled the virtues of cocaine as a stimulant and innocent producer of euphoria. They also proclaimed it perfectly safe.

By 1905 when its use peaked, the dangers of cocaine—in particular, its production of paranoid delusions and its contribution to violent crime—were becoming apparent. An aroused public came to fear the "drug fiend" and supported restrictive legislation. The public seems to be approaching a similar state of awareness today, as the cocaine epidemic exacts an increasingly fearsome toll in all social strata, especially the lower ones.

Amphetamines were not developed until 1936 but they had an immediate impact. The pattern of their reception duplicated in many respects that of cocaine. From the start the drug was extolled as a stimulant, a producer of euphoria, and a source of improved athletic and intellectual performance. Medical authorities pronounced it safe and prescribed huge amounts for depression, morphine addiction, seasickness, heart block, and excessive weight, among many other "indications." Inhalants containing amphetamine were available without prescription. All of the major belligerents in World War II issued amphetamines to their armed forces. Adolf Hitler is very likely to have used the drug freely both intravenously and by mouth, and it probably contributed to his army's defeat at Stalingrad and to some subsequent disasters suffered by his military forces. But it was not until huge stores of methamphetamine that the Japanese military had stockpiled during the war reached illegal markets in Japan and North America and produced a major epidemic that the dangers of the drug became too apparent to ignore. Laws and regulations followed, but it was an informed and aroused public that made enforcement feasible.

In recent years, crack has been the focus of much of the public concern with abuse of stimulants. Crack is perhaps the most addicting drug known with respect to drug seeking. After a few episodes of smoking crack, craving for the drug is described as so great that users will do anything to get it. Moreover, the rapidity of onset is accompanied by short duration of action—10 to 30 minutes—so multiple administration over a period of use is the rule. Crack's toxicity features hypervigilant excitement and paranoia, a potentially lethal coupling that often leads to physical confrontations resulting in injury or death. Because the cost of crack is great and the user's addiction to the drug is extreme, crack use often breeds crime. Among males arrested for non-drug-related felony offenses, large proportions have cocaine in urine samples (ranging, in one study, from 78 percent in New York City to 38 percent in San Antonio).

Tolerance and Withdrawal

Tolerance to the euphoric effect of stimulants leads to increased total daily dosage, in this case mainly because of more frequent administration of about the same dose, rather than increased size of individual doses. Tolerance to other drug effects (appetite suppression in particular) also comes about.

Stimulant drugs do not produce dependence or withdrawal marked by measurable physical discomfort; there is no direct physiologic threat to life, as there is in the withdrawal of sedatives. However, withdrawal leads to profound depression and to desperate seeking of the drug. If no drug is available, the depression can result in suicide.

Treatment

Treatment for stimulant abuse amounts to encouraging abstinence from the drug, and success is gauged by the length of the abstinent periods. Use of crack, in particular, must be seen as a chronic relapsing disease. Drug-free intervals, not permanent abstinence, are the realistic goal of treatment. Recently, researchers have begun using antidepressant drugs to counter the profound depression associated with stimulant withdrawal. This new departure is based on a reasonable pharmacologic rationale. Because stimulants increase the amount of dopamine in the synaptic cleft, prolonged use would presumably exhaust dopamine stores in the vesicles of transmitting neurons, which would leave insufficient dopamine available to the brain's normal reward system. Antidepressant drugs inhibit reuptake of dopamine, which might, as a consequence, sustain dopamine stimulation until a natural balance could be re-established. So far, the results of this treatment approach are promising but inconclusive.

Hallucinogenic Drugs

Drugs in the hallucinogenic class have many different chemical structures and act by several different mechanisms. But the effect they all can produce which is sought by users is distortions of sensory input. The distortions may involve shape, color, taste, touch, or position in space. Ordinary objects may appear much larger or smaller than they really are, and they may have fluid, shifting outlines and vivid, changing coloration. Sometimes objects seem highlighted, sometimes more distant. Users report hearing music differently; it seems to be clearer, more sharply focused, and meaningful in new and subtle ways. Time does not proceed evenly. These distorted experiences may seem charged with meaning, yielding irreplaceable insights into the nature of life and the cosmos. New, sometimes radically different meanings seem to emerge out of common experiences. Sometimes the sensory experience is associated with intense fear or rage—a "bad trip"—which all too often leads to catastrophic behavior. The effects of these drugs are very hard to predict. They vary with the personality of the user, with the user's current mood and physical condition, and, most important, with the environment in which the drugs are taken.

The dominant sensory experiences associated with hallucinogenic drugs are not hallucinations at all. They are better described as *illusions*, because most of them are obviously related to actual objects or events in the user's environment. (True hallucinations have little or no basis in sensory input from the environment.) However, the illusions are unusually graphic ones, and they are associated with unusually intense feeling states.

The most important of the hallucinogenic drugs are *LSD* (*lysergic acid*), *PCP* (*phencyclidine*), *marijuana*, and several types of *inhalants*, mainly hydrocarbons. As these drugs are used by humans, tolerance to them does not develop, and withdrawal produces no serious disturbances. Whether or not they are reinforcing seems to depend mainly on the personality of the user. Prolonged use of inhalants, LSD, or phencyclidine produces permanent changes in the brain. Marijuana is probably not permanently damaging to the brain in ordinary use, but it may do permanent damage if used intensively for several years.

LSD

The effects of LSD are similar to those of mescaline and peyote, but LSD is a synthetic compound effective in extremely small doses, whereas the other two are natural plant products. LSD acts on the serotonin receptors of nerve cells first to stimulate, later to inhibit, the receptor and hence the cell. Although the effects of an average dose persist a relatively long time—about 8 hours—users may be troubled—even incapacitated—by flashbacks that appear long after ingestion of the drug. Flashbacks consist of vivid relivings of the sensory and emotional experiences of a "trip," usually a bad trip. Flashbacks may come at any time, without warning, and can be highly disruptive. Flashbacks diminish in frequency over time but may recur periodically, with terrifying intensity, for years.

Flashbacks, or closely related phenomena, are also associated with other drugs. Drug paraphernalia (such as needles or spoons) may trigger intense reliving of a past drug experience. Odd associations may develop; for example, paper money seems to trigger intense desire for drug in some cocaine users. Former tobacco smokers report similar states when they describe intense craving triggered by a whiff of tobacco or by the sight of someone smoking.

PCP

Also known as "dust" and "angel dust," PCP, an anesthetic drug that was widely used in veterinary medicine, came briefly into vogue during the the 1970s. But it soon became known as so dangerous that it fell from favor. Recently, however, PCP has apparently staged an alarming comeback; it is smoked with cocaine in a preparation known as space balls. In Washington, D.C., all persons arrested for felonies are administered tests for drugs. In 1986, 60.3 percent of those so arrested had used PCP or cocaine or both. Of those, about a third had used PCP alone. In that year the city's emergency rooms recorded a 280 percent increase in PCP-related visits.

PCP interferes with neurotransmission through the neurotransmitter glutamic acid, but the exact mechanism of action is unknown. This powerful hallucinogenic drug produces distortions in the user's perception of the environment that are unusually frightening, bizarre, and persistent. The acute effects last several hours, but other effects (including apathy and an apparent emotional blunting that resembles chronic schizophrenia) may persist much longer.

Inhalants

Antifreeze, gasoline, paint thinner, glues, shoe polish, room deodorants—all these and many other substances have been used as inhalants. The effects on the human brain are cruder than those of other hallucinogens, but then inhalants are cheaper and more readily available. According to professionals who deal with users, damage to the brain over time is severe, but it is hard to define because the users tend to be ghetto or barrio youngsters who soon graduate to other drugs, making it uncertain both when damage occurred and just what caused it. Hearing loss is certain. Loss of intellectual capacity is almost certain.

Marijuana

Marijuana is the most commonly used of the hallucinogenic drugs. Demand for it is so great that it is one of this country's major cash crops. Indeed, American growers have become so proficient at raising large quantities of high-quality product that marijuana is now an export crop that is much prized by the more sophisticated of foreign users. Our agricultural genius again strikes at the trade deficit.

The potency of different marijuana preparations varies widely. Marijuana is the dried leaf of the hemp plant, which has an average concentration of psychoactive ingredients of about 1 percent by weight. Historically, this concentration was much less, but presumably because of scientific agriculture, it has been increasing recently: Some samples have attained 3 to 4 percent. Cannabis is a generic term for all preparations containing active drug, but it is generally applied only to preparations more potent than dried leaf. The most potent form of cannabis, known as hashish, is prepared by scraping the dried resin from the leaves of especially potent plants.

The effect of cannabis depends on the strength of the preparation used. Hashish's effect is comparable to that of any other hallucinogenic drug while low-potency preparations produce milder effects. Users describe the sought-after effect as an intensely pleasant, relaxed, dreamy state. Perceptions are not physically distorted but seem to take on pleasurable meanings. While a person is so intoxicated, his or her driving and fine coordination are impaired. In rare instances, disabling anxiety and depression follow the hallucinogenic experience.

The use of marijuana over a long period of time is associated with an unmotivated state. Whether this apathy is produced by marijuana itself or by other factors characteristic of the lifestyles of chronic users is unclear. Whatever the cause, some marijuana users lack ambition and initiative, neglect their appearance, and seem intellectually dulled. They tend to change their residence frequently and are prone to depressions and to engaging in impulsive, destructive acts. They become chronic failures in school, personal relationships, and work.

Treatment

There is no specific treatment for users of hallucinogenic drugs. Because these drugs do not produce tolerance, no medical treatment is needed for withdrawal. Abstinence is the only possible treatment, and in today's society, that must be voluntary. There is no serious possibility that enforcing laws could keep these drugs out of the hands of people who want them.

Narcotics

The narcotic, or opiate, drugs include several products of the opium poppy—mainly opium, heroin, morphine, and codeine—and such synthetic narcotics as Demerol (meperidine). Narcotic drugs were also prominent in the drug abuse epidemic of the late nineteenth and early twentieth centuries. Morphine was purified from crude extract of the opium poppy in 1806, and soon thereafter chemists learned how to convert morphine into heroin. These narcotics were freely sold in drugstores, as were hypodermic needles, which conveniently had been invented at about the same time. Morphine was so widely used in the American Civil War that morphine addiction became known as soldier's disease. Public reaction against narcotics merged with the reaction against cocaine; as a result, both were included in the Harrison Anti-Narcotic Act of 1914.

Tolerance and Withdrawal

Narcotics characteristically produce a dreamy, relaxed euphoria in experienced users. They are powerfully reinforcing. Perception of pain is greatly lessened, which is the main reason for their legitimate medical use. Tolerance develops to several effects, especially pain relief and euphoria. Despite the depictions in movies, withdrawal is only uncomfortable, not life-threatening. About 8 to 12 hours after the last dose, the withdrawing addict exhibits tearing and a runny nose and then falls into a restless sleep (the "yen") for another 8 to 12 hours. By 60 to 72 hours after the last dose, distress is at its high point. It is marked by restlessness, irritability, sleeplessness, severe sneezing, weakness, depressed mood, shaking chills, abdominal cramps, and diarrhea. Over the next week, these signs diminish and then cease. But it now appears that full physiologic restitution to a pre-addicted state in *any* addiction, including one to narcotics, may take years.

Exposure to narcotics is necessary to produce self-destructive addiction, but it is only one element in the chain and is not sufficient in itself. This is dramatically illustrated by a footnote to America's Vietnam war experience. Heroin was readily available in Vietnam and was widely used by American service personnel. Yet most users, though addicted, stopped using narcotics almost immediately when they returned to this country. They endured a few days of discomfort in withdrawal and never looked back. A small minority, mainly those who returned to ghetto conditions, persisted in using narcotics. (See the L. Robins volume cited in the readings for this chapter in Appendix A.)

It has long been known that many users—mainly people in the middle and often professional classes—have injected narcotics for years without demonstrable ill effect on their health or economic productivity. Clearly, more than drug availability is involved in our present epidemic. The "pusher" who provides drugs is one essential link. But also at work is a complex of social and cultural factors that are far from understood.

Intravenous Drugs and AIDS

In addition to the long-recognized and well-known consequences of intravenous drug abuse, a further life-threatening danger has emerged in recent years: AIDS. *Acquired immune deficiency syndrome (AIDS)* is rampant among the 1.1 to 1.3 million U.S. intravenous (IV) drug abusers. Forty-two thousand of them have developed the full disease or have already died from it; they represent about 30 percent of the 140,000 total American victims. Estimates of the rate of seropositivity (exhibited by those who are infected with the virus but have not yet the developed the full-blown disease) among IV drug abusers are in the range of 20 percent nationwide. In New York City, the first and most heavily infected city, more than 60 percent of intravenous drug abusers who seek treatment are seropositive. The proportion is lower in other cities, but it is rising in a pattern that threatens to duplicate New York's experience. Moreover, infection is expanding outward from the drug users themselves to their sexual partners and to their newborn children. In Box 6, other effects of drug abuse on the unborn are described.

Transmission of the AIDS virus among intravenous drug users occurs through shared hypodermic needles, syringes, and other items of drug paraphernalia. Whether in "shooting galleries" that may service dozens of users, or among smaller groups in rooms or back alleys, needles and syringes are in chronic short supply. Both are actually rented in some localities. An addict may inject several times a day for several days, and equipment is used over and over again. Transmission is also boosted by certain rituals of injection. Users prolong the actual injection of drug by repeatedly drawing blood up into the syringe and injecting it back into the vein. This heightens the anticipation and prolongs the pleasure of the actual drug effect. It also gives the virus added deadly chances to spread.

A huge education campaign has been mounted to warn the drug-using population about the dangers of sharing equipment and to attempt to enroll as many users as possible in treatment programs. However, after 4 years of intensive effort, about 70 percent of IV users still acknowledge sharing needles. This figure improves to about 50 percent in specific populations after they have been targeted by a major educative effort. Public-policy options that once seemed radical, such as providing free needles, are now being tried. But intravenous drug users are a very difficult population to reach, and the logistics of making free needles easily available in cities with a large underclass have not been worked out.

Box 5   Drug Abuse and the Newborn

It is surprising that none of the drugs considered in this chapter has yet been proved to harm unborn children permanently. This is because the evidence, though plentiful, is not conclusive. For example, marijuana probably affects fetal development adversely. A fetal marijuana syndrome has been described that resembles the fetal alcohol syndrome outlined in Chapter 6 and is associated with permanent damage. Newborns addicted to narcotics and "crack babies" are well known to hospital nursery personnel. The addicted child often has to go through withdrawal just like an adult. Crack babies are hyperactive and easily startled. The follow-up studies needed to estimate the long-term outcome for such children are still under way, but it is clear that they tend to be underweight and to develop slowly. However, uncertainty persists about the causes of the poor start that children of drug-abusing mothers get. The mother is usually an unmarried, unemployed adolescent who has had no prenatal care, has used several different drugs during the pregnancy, has had an inadequate diet, and then presents herself to an emergency room just in time to deliver an underweight infant two months prematurely. Such children probably have a bleak future—but not just for one reason. The whole deck has been stacked against them.

Treatment

At present, the single narcotic treatment program that has proved effective in the addicted population is methadone maintenance. Results improve when intensive vocational and social counseling is combined with methadone in a comprehensive program.

Methadone is itself a narcotic drug. It occupies morphine receptors in the brain and can substitute for morphine in preventing withdrawal (see Box 7). The great advantages of methadone are that it has a long period of action—a full day—and that it is active when taken by mouth. It also produces less euphoria than most other narcotics. In treatment programs, enough methadone is given to saturate the brain's receptors. Therefore, if another narcotic is taken after methadone, it does not produce euphoria. Because a daily dose prevents craving for the drug, drug seeking ceases to dominate an

---

Box 6   Narcotic Drugs and the Brain

Over the last few years, scientific understanding of narcotics has been revolutionized by the discovery of the receptors in brain tissue that are affected by narcotic drugs and of the natural substances that normally occupy them. The logic underlying the research that led to these discoveries is fascinating.

It seemed obvious to pharmacologists that such substances as heroin and morphine must be mimicking the action on brain tissue of naturally occurring chemicals, probably those which relieved pain. Moreover, they thought, that action must be based on nerve-cell receptor molecules similar to those acted on by natural neurotransmitters. With the development of specific radioactive chemicals that could be used as tracers, the hunt was on. Radioactive morphine was used to locate areas in the brain where

(Continued)

(Box 6 continued)

morphine became attached to naturally occurring receptor molecules.

Once the morphine receptors were located, it became feasible to search for natural chemicals that occupied them. Soon the search was rewarded. A substance with morphine-like action was isolated and named *enkephalin*. It was quickly learned that enkephalin acts in nature to prevent or lessen pain; it is a substance produced by the body that has opiate properties. Following the same rationale, several other naturally occurring substances that influence the function of nerve cells have been discovered, and more are under investigation.

The discovery of morphine receptors also made it possible to design specific molecules that would occupy some of the same receptor molecules that morphine occupies. In this way, drugs that had some of the properties of narcotics, but not others, were invented. As we noted earlier, other drugs have been designed that occupy these receptors for long periods of time, thus blocking them and preventing narcotic drugs from acting. This line of research has led to new treatment options, and though none has yet proved effective, promising leads continue to be actively investigated.

addict's life. In fact, a daily dose of methadone is compatible with normal working and social life.

Because it sustains rather than cures the basic addiction, methadone is far from an ideal answer. Though not so powerfully reinforcing as morphine or heroin, it can prevent withdrawal symptoms and is hence a prized street drug. Huge quantities of methadone have been diverted from treatment clinics to the street trade. Considerable effort has gone into using methadone as one stage in progressive total withdrawal of narcotics. For example, methadone might be substituted for heroin and then be itself withdrawn. This plan of treatment is sometimes effective, though not for large numbers of addicts.

Other treatments are based on newer drugs that block narcotic receptors but that, unlike methadone, have no narcotic action. Attempts have been made to substitute these drugs either for methadone, or directly for a street narcotic. The theory is that when the receptor is blocked, street drugs, if used, will have no effect. So far, these treatment programs have not proved effective.

What to Do About Drug Abuse?

To individuals coming to grips with drug abuse of their own or in their families, and, in fact, to all members of our society, drugs present a huge problem—but not an insurmountable one.

■ *If You Are Abusing Drugs*

You have surely tried to quit by yourself—not just once but several times—and have failed. You will have to reach two conclusions about your problem before you have much chance of dealing with it. First, you must decide that drug abuse is having such severe adverse effects on your life that you must stop. Second, you must accept that you cannot stop alone. When you are ready to address your problem, there are a variety of treatment programs available. Get into one. But understand that you are still the one who will have to undergo the discomfort of stopping the use of drugs. Don't expect to have an easy time. Treatment will mainly consist of stripping away all of your excuses and rationalizations and helping you rearrange your attitudes so that they are compatible with a drug-free life. It's going to be tough, but it's going to be worth it.

■ *If Someone Close to You Is Abusing Drugs*

Over many generations, a few do's and don'ts have proved important.

• Do decide whether drugs really are a problem that needs corrective action. Is drug use threatening health or important vocational, personal, or family goals? If it is, and if you decide to act, you must be resolute. Half-way measures will make things worse.

• Don't be swayed by your personal moral values when answering this question for a relative. Remember that people vary greatly in their ability to manage drugs (alcohol in particular) without significant ill effects. Be sure your action is really needed before you proceed further.

• Do learn the facts about any drug that seems to present a problem. Several sources of information are listed in Appendix A.

• Don't preach, nag, weep, plead, threaten, or convey moral superiority. Patiently tell the user why you think a problem exists that must be addressed. Drug abusers can offer unlimited excuses and rationalizations. Be prepared for these, and stick to your carefully thought-out plan.

• Do insist on obtaining medical evaluation and treatment if you think it is needed, and observe simple precautions such as not allowing an intoxicated person to drive.

• Don't yield on the need for treatment. If you must give an ultimatum—treatment or else—be sure that you follow through, even if this means separation or judicial commitment.

• Do be positive about those attributes of the user that you admire and expect will be even more valuable when drug abuse is controlled.

• Your only target is drug abuse. Don't deviate from that goal because of promises of other behavioral reforms. If drug use is not stopped, such promises are most unlikely to be kept anyway.

■ *What to Do About Drugs as a Member of Society*

Obviously, drug abuse is a serious problem in the Western industrial democracies as well as in much of the rest of the world. How can we best approach this problem? Attempts to reduce the supply of illegal drugs entering this country have proved ineffective. It is simply impossible to police our borders so thoroughly that any significant proportion of the incoming supply is stopped. In early 1991, the cost of cocaine on the U.S. market was $21,000 to $30,000 per kilogram. This is up about 50 percent from 1989, so it is reasonable to conclude that current intensive efforts at interdiction are having some effect, but only a moderate one. On the other hand, making drugs freely available increases the rate of addiction while doing little to curb illicit drug use. We should not open our borders, and we should make things as difficult as possible for traffickers, but we cannot expect cutting down on the supply to yield conclusive results.

The best way to decrease the supply of drugs in this country is to reduce the demand for them through public education. This is what controlled the first cocaine and narcotics epidemic in the early decades of this century. Today it is slowly reducing use of nicotine, an extremely addicting drug.

Today's educational efforts are focused on illegally imported drugs, especially cocaine, but there is every reason to expand them to include other classes of drugs. Special subgroups might be targeted for special effort. For example, it has been shown that children of alcoholics run about four times as much risk of developing major problems with alcohol as children of non-alcoholics. Such high-risk children might well benefit from educational experiences aimed at teaching them the early signs of addictive alcoholism. Julia discovered these on her own, and in somewhat different circumstances, she might have avoided major problems in her life. As it was, she behaved for many years as though alcohol were a special hazard for her, and during those years she established herself in adult life. When problems finally 0did develop, she had educational, social, and financial resources. Her relatively good outcome is probably attributable in part to those resources, coupled with her early self-education. This model could be widely and systematically applied.

Part

5

BEHAVIOR

...

Many of the people who seek out a psychiatrist on their own, and even more of those who are sent to one, have no definable, consistent problem with mood or thinking or any other mental process, and no structural changes have occurred in their brains. Even so, their behavior becomes erratic and severely disordered from time to time. Such people are said to have a *personality disorder*, or *behavior disorder*. It is important that only sometimes is their behavior problematic. Often they can effectively control their actions, and when they do, their behavior is socially acceptable, even constructive. Months can pass without problems. But unpredictably, an apparently impulsive, senseless, self-defeating, or antisocial act will trigger conflict with those around them or with society in general. Such people do not usually regard themselves as ill: they complain of no symptoms, no dis-ease. Whether some yet-undiscovered biochemical or tissue pathology underlies the behavior disorders has been argued for decades. Medicine can only say that we all have destructive impulses that most of us manage to control, and that despite intensive searches, there is no evidence that failure to control them can be associated with illness.

The designation *personality disorder* has been applied to a multitude of behavior patterns that have been considered deviant at different times in different societies. Chapter 8 describes the most socially disruptive of these patterns, the one associated with criminality. Then, following the trail marked by the clustering of illnesses within families (see Box 3 on page ooo), it goes on to consider mental disorders marked by widespread somatic (bodily) symptoms. The validity of several other constructs in the diagnostic nomenclature, such as "passive-aggressive personality" is weakly supported by evidence, and such categories will not be considered separately.

Several intense professional and societal controversies surround the disorders associated with sexuality, which are described in Chapter 9. In this respect, some of the same issues arise as with the behavior disorders: Is a medical diagnosis warranted? What societal sanctions are appropriate for which behaviors? Should social controls be imposed over behaviors associated with sexually transmitted diseases? Thus sexual disorders seem to belong in this section, although the fit is imperfect.

8

Antisocial Personality and Somatoform Disorder

□ □ □

❏ *Roger*

Roger had always said he was born cursed. In fact, he was the second child born to the first marriage of each of his parents. When Roger was a child, his mother worked off and on as a waitress but was actually at home ill much of the time. She was a cheerful, overweight woman who complained regularly about assorted aches and pains, especially incapacitating headaches and menstrual distress. Sometimes she had seizures during which she would writhe on the floor for several minutes and after which she seemed confused. Twice she was paralyzed from the waist down after a seizure, but she recovered over a couple of days. By age 25 she had had five operations on her sexual organs: four D & C's, and, finally, a hysterectomy. Over the next five years she lost her appendix and gall bladder and had two operations to undo ad- hesions caused by earlier operations. No causes were ever found for her many medical troubles. But despite all of this she was a gregarious, cheerful woman who loved to chat with neighbors and, given the slightest encouragement, would describe her operations in dramatic detail.

Roger's father was a long-distance truck driver who was often in trouble with police, creditors, and licensing authorities. Several times he was charged with battery or assault stemming from fights, usually in bars. But he drove his truck hard and steadily and brought home a good income.

Roger's mother and father were divorced shortly after he was born. His father had several times beaten his mother because she found sex painful or distasteful, but after the divorce their relationship was cordial. He was soon remarried to a cousin of Roger's mother and, with his new wife, settled in the same neighborhood. Within five years Roger had three half-sisters. The extended families were in frequent social contact, and Roger divided his days and nights between the two homes as his whims led him.

Roger did not respond well to school. By the sixth grade, he had been suspended twice for fighting and had often been truant. He had turned out to be a handsome child, always neatly dressed, with a winning personality. He was also well above average in intelligence, which made his teachers especially eager to help and especially frustrated when they failed to do so. He attributed his troubles to his parent's divorce and to worries about his mother's illnesses. He was very convincing as he described his plight, and his promises to reform were accepted.

In the seventh grade, his police record began. Then age 14, he was apprehended twice for stealing bicycles and once for shoplifting. He also had begun drinking alcohol and smoking, and he claimed he had used LSD and "speed" (amphetamine). The juvenile authorities didn't know whether to believe he was really using drugs, but because of the thefts, truancy, and fighting, he was placed in a foster home. He promptly ran away and was placed in another foster home, where he lasted two weeks before running away with his foster mother's jewelry in his pocket and a color television strapped to his bicycle. He was sent to a reform school.

There Roger became interested in both auto mechanics and the machine shop. He was quick to learn and turned out neat, accurate work. Although he was disciplined several times for not doing his chores and for breaking rules, he did fairly well at the school, and nine months after his arrival, he was being considered for discharge to his father's home. He maintained that his father's rough and strict discipline was what he needed in order to reform his life. His counselors were ready to agree, but just a week before his release, he assaulted a cottage-mate, inflicting a broken jaw and a concussion. The assault was judged to be an impulsive act mounted without provocation or warning. Roger was transferred to an adult prison, where he spent the next six months.

When he was released, Roger went to his father's home. He started back to school but soon dropped out. After that he worked irregularly in service stations and seasonally in a cannery, but mostly he just hung out with one or more of a casual group of half a dozen youths. They spent most of their time obtaining beer and drugs, which they took to the home of one of their number or, in good weather, to an isolated bluff overlooking a river.

One summer evening Roger and another boy were out riding their bicycles looking for something to do. They met a young man, took him to the home of Roger's sister, who was away, and, in the basement, beat him to death by kicking and hitting with a baseball bat. They maintained that they were trying to defend themselves against homosexual advances and grew so angry that they became temporarily insane. The state, however, proved that their motive was robbery, and Roger was convicted of murder. Before sentencing, he confessed to robbery but told the prosecuting attorney that his accomplice was the instigator of the crime and did the actual killing. At the same time he was writing notes to his accomplice that were intercepted by the jailors. In these notes Roger promised to remain silent, begged his accomplice to admit nothing, and pledged eternal friendship. Then barely 16, he was again sentenced to a juvenile correction facility. Statutes governing juvenile crime in his state mandated his release at age 19.

For a year after his release, only a bad-check charge, the theft of a case of beer, and fighting marred Roger's legal record. He worked for several months at a steel supplier but was fired after an argument. For a short time he worked as a lifeguard; he even became a minor local hero by pulling an exhausted and possibly drowning child from the municipal pool. Finally, his father managed to get him hired by a trucking company.

By then Roger was living with his older sister and her husband, a stable couple who maintained a stable home. They had two children, whom Roger seemed to adore. His sister sympathized with him and attributed much of his trouble to his father. Roger had also become friendly with his cousin's family, who lived nearby. His cousin was married to a man who had several children by other marriages. One child, a 17-year-old daughter, was still at home. Roger began dating her, and after she became pregnant, they married.

Roger's work as a truck driver seemed to suit him. However, his life remained troubled. There were occasional barroom fights, and once the police were highly suspicious that he had beaten another man to death. A partly decomposed male body was found in a river near where Roger lived; an autopsy discovered several fractures, including a massive skull injury. The victim was a known homosexual who had been seen with Roger. The police questioned Roger but did not find enough evidence to proceed against him. Problems also developed between Roger and his sister who finally ordered him never again to set foot in her home. And his marriage disintegrated. His wife had come to fear him and had called the police several times because of domestic violence. She was desperate. During one of Roger's trucking trips, she took their son and moved to another state, where she had relatives. Roger appeared distraught when he discovered that his wife had left him, but either no one knew where she had gone or no one would admit to knowing.

For several months Roger continued to work and lived much as he had before his wife left. He became emotional when he described loving and missing his wife and son. But he did little about it and began staying with another woman. Then he was arrested again, this time for stealing new automobile tires from a delivery truck. Roger and the driver of the truck had been drinking together through a long lunch break. At his next delivery, the driver found that 20 tires were missing. Roger had no defense; 4

of the tires were found on his girlfriend's automobile. He was sentenced to 6 months in the county workhouse and actually served 100 days.

Roger was not seen for several days after his release from the workhouse. He next appeared at the home of his wife's parents. His mother-in-law, then age 50, worked cleaning rooms at a motel. Her husband, 10 years older, was incapacitated by heart and lung disease. They knew Roger well. Later she told the police that at first she and her husband had liked him, that "he could tell great stories and be a lot of fun." But within a short time, they had seen his other sides. He was not a welcome guest, but when he appeared at their door, the couple admitted him to their home. After unsuccessful attempts to get his in-laws to contact their daughter, Roger abruptly said, "You know I'm sorry to have to do this." Taking out a knife, he forced both of them into the basement. He tied the husband to a chair, then took his mother-in-law with him while he ransacked the house. In an upstairs bedroom, he raped her. Afterward he took her back to the basement, tied her, and took her husband upstairs. She heard them drive off. An hour later the automobile returned and Roger reappeared. "Your husband is safe, but he is tied up where no one will find him unless I tell them where to go," he said. "You had better cooperate." In fact, her husband was already dead. Roger had beaten him to death with a tire iron and hidden his body in the trunk of an automobile parked in a wrecking yard.

For four days Roger kept his mother-in-law prisoner, raping her repeatedly. The end of her ordeal came on an excursion to buy groceries. Roger had parked the automobile in the parking lot of a large motel so he could go into the bar and drink. She was left in the car, deadly afraid that if she ran to get police help, Roger would escape and would never reveal where her husband was being held. But he had parked the car at a remote location in the parking lot, where it attracted the attention of a security guard. The guard approached the car and soon had the whole story. Roger was apprehended without a struggle. He was sentenced to death but at this writing has not been executed.

Diagnosis: Antisocial Personality

Roger's diagnosis was antisocial personality. About 4 percent of adult American males and 1 percent of females meet the diagnostic criteria for this condition. These include onset by age 15 and persistence for at least 3 years of such behaviors as truancy, expulsion from school, under-achievement in school, thefts, running away, persistent lying, sexual promiscuity, vandalism, and fighting. In adults, antisocial personality is marked by a failure to adapt to working on a consistent and responsible basis, irresponsible parenting, inability to maintain an enduring sexual attachment, criminal activity, irritability, physical aggressiveness, impulsivity, lying to or "conning" others, and reckless disregard of the safety of oneself or others. Often, though not always, these behaviors are paired with a bright and charming personality. Many antisocial persons are great con artists. Roger fits the diagnosis in every respect.

Antisocial personality, like other so-called personality disorders, is not marked by any consistent disorder of thinking, perception, or mood. Affected people are in full command of their behavior in that there is no defect of reasoning or any other measurable mental attribute that might make destructive behaviors more probable. Moreover, they do not regard themselves as ill, and it was only in the middle of this century that the possibility of illness was raised. Those who believed that illness is behind such personalities reasoned that something clearly is wrong with people like Roger who at times, and for no apparent reason, behave in such irrational, self-defeating ways. This behavior must be the result of an illness that we cannot now define in terms of attributes such as thinking or mood, but an illness nevertheless. When optimism over psychiatric treatment was at its peak just after World War II, this view became the predominant one in American psychiatry. (The rest of the world was much slower to accept it and has even now not done so completely.)

Prognosis

The prognosis for antisocial personality is not promising. It has long been part of professional lore that antisocials tend to become more tractable after about age 30. However, if this occurs, it may be a general consequence of age rather than an improvement in the basic condition.

Treatment

There is no recognized treatment for such persons. Strict supervision on parole, where the consequences of problem behavior are made unmistakably clear and follow through is certain, does appear to help prevent criminal recidivism. Most attempts at more active treatment have involved group therapy, a treatment effort that began after World War II with discharged soldier-offenders. It was found that groups of antisocials did tend to control their members as long as such groups stayed together. Permanent behavior change was not demonstrated. However, the initial results seemed promising, and this promise, added to the optimism of the period, led judges, attorneys, and juries indiscriminately to accept antisocials as mentally ill and treatable. Many were committed to mental hospitals. This came about mainly because of a sincere desire to help. But in addition, prosecuting authorities learned that committing criminals to mental hospitals often took them off the street longer than sentencing them to penal institutions.

Much of the confusion that resulted is only now being resolved. Although many antisocials remain in the mental health system, psychiatrists no longer believe they have a credible theory of antisocial behavior, much less know how to treat it successfully, and the criminal justice system has become more realistic about the prognosis for antisocial persons. However, a price is being paid. Genuinely ill persons (such as those with schizophrenia) who have performed a criminal act while affected by a delusion or another mental aberration and who were once absolved by law from responsibility for their actions, are now increasingly being handled by the criminal justice system. What to do about these persons is a major problem for psychiatry, the law, and society.

■ The Insanity Defense ■

In 1843 Daniel M'Naghten, an insane man, was charged with murder. The defense invoked M'Naghten's obvious insanity, which eventually resulted in the English House of Lords promulgating the famous M'Naghten rules. These rules state that in order to escape responsibility for a criminal act, the accused person must have had, at the time of the criminal act, a defect of reason resulting from "disease of the mind, so as not to know the nature and quality of the act, or if he did know it, not to know that what he was doing was wrong." Despite repeated attempts to modify these standards or do away with them altogether, today they generally govern the insanity defense in American courts.

In theory there are two distinct phases of the legal processes involving criminal behavior and insanity. First, the examining expert (usually a psychiatrist) is asked to determine whether the defendant is capable of standing trial. Does the defendant understand the crime with which she or he is charged and the possible outcomes of a trial on those charges? Can he or she comprehend an oath to tell the truth and the penalty for perjury? Is the defendant capable of cooperating with court processes and with attorneys? Only severely ill persons fail these tests and are judged unfit to stand trial. They are then held in a hospital until they are fit. The second phase is submission of the M'Naghten questions to a jury in the form of a judge's instructions. The jury will have observed the defendant and will have heard evidence relating to the crime, as well as testimony (probably conflicting) from experts. The members of the jury must decide whether the offense is excusable because of insanity.

In practice, matters are usually handled more pragmatically. Minor offenses are generally disposed of without a trial. Judges, with or without psychiatric advice, may commit an accused person to a mental hospital and so bypass formal trial. Often the first and second phases we have noted are merged. Judges ask for and receive informal opinions from psychiatrists about the applicability of M'Naghten rules to a case at the time when, strictly speaking, only competence to stand trial should be in question. These practical procedures are generally fair when applied to routine problems. It is the more serious, or (worse) the more sensational cases wherein justice is sometimes compromised.

Why does the justice system seem so unsatisfactory when the insanity defense is invoked in major crimes? To lay people, it often appears that murderers, rapists, and switchblade artists are loosed on the community by feather-headed shrinks and bleeding-heart judges. In fact, few persons successfully invoke an insanity defense, and those who do go to prison–hospitals where they remain for relatively long periods.

Within the prison hospitals, successful treatment can present the professionals charged with custodial responsibility with uncomfortable dilemmas. Many psychiatric illnesses can be treated so quickly and successfully that an ill person who has committed a crime may be unrecognizable a few weeks later. Other cases require longer periods of treatment, but many offenders become mentally stable sooner or later, and it is difficult for hospital personnel to accept responsibility for people who would be quickly discharged from care were it not for their criminal acts. Decisions about subsequent management are not self-evident, however. Treatment usually includes ongoing medical supervision and the taking of therapeutic drugs. Enforcement of these requirements involves methods that medicine is neither equipped for nor inclined to adopt. These considerations have led many states to appoint review panels consisting typically of attorneys, mental health professionals, and lay persons that are charged with supervising released offenders. The offender and the hospital that has custody develop a plan consisting of graded steps toward full discharge. Such plans usually require medical supervision, a job, and a structured living arrangement. The review body examines the plan and, if it finds it practical, supervises its implementation through a process much like probation (though probably stricter overall).

Despite these safeguards, the public remains most dissatisfied with the courts' handling of mentally ill offenders. To appreciate the problems, consider what the criminal justice system is supposed to accomplish by incarcerating criminals. There are four broadly recognized aims:

1. Prevention of crime, thus safeguarding the public. When they are locked away, criminals cannot commit crimes.

2. Reform (or rehabilitation). While locked away, criminals will learn the error of their ways and may also master useful skills.

3. Deterrence. Locking criminals away causes potential criminals to think again before breaking the law.

4. Revenge. Society should punish the criminal to a degree consistent with the crime committed. "An eye for an eye."

Evidence shows that incarceration actually achieves only the first of these aims. The other aims may fit various personal and social agendas, but they are seldom achieved—or even advanced—by incarceration. There is no evidence that incarceration promotes rehabilitation. If anything, the evidence suggests that prison turns many people into hardened and more skillful criminals. Moreover, there is no evidence that rehabilitation can be systematically achieved by any other means, though there are hints that tough, no-nonsense parole, with certain return to prison as an immediate consequence of any violation may help control overt criminal behavior. Deterrence may be effective in a limited range of crimes, such as cheating on income tax returns, but otherwise, criminals are not deterred by examples made of other criminals. Finally, criminals don't generally feel punished. Society may feel that it punishes, but those we "punish" most often feel wronged, believe they are victims of forces beyond their control, or are indifferent to the whole process. On the other hand, that incarceration accomplishes the first aim is self-evident. A criminal cannot offend against the larger society while locked away. That is an important result, because there can be no doubt that such safeguarding is needed. It alone can justify incarceration, and it is justification enough.

■■■

How should we, as a society, respond to criminal offenses committed by mentally ill persons? To answer sensibly, we must first acknowledge that neither psychiatrists nor other mental health professionals can predict violent or criminal behavior any more accurately than lay persons. The evidence relied on by professionals and lay persons alike is past history of violent or uncontrolled behavior, and both find the same inescapable conclusion when they interpret the evidence: Such behavior is likely to be repeated. What, then, should society do? I think that neither psychiatry nor any other behavior science has good answers. The first aim of incarceration, safeguarding the public, is as applicable to the mentally ill as to the purely antisocial. As in criminal law generally, juries, well informed by competent and responsible experts, offer the best hope for sensible and humane decisions about how society should deal with ill persons who commit criminal acts. I personally feel that one who has performed a violent criminal act such as murder, whether ill or not, has crossed a threshold beyond which the rights of society have priority over the rights of the criminal. No one can accurately predict whether such an individual would kill again if given provocation and opportunity. What we *can* say that such a person is more likely kill than a person who has never killed—an unsatisfying conclusion but one that should carry great weight.

Psychiatric Illness Mimicking General Medical Illness

Roger was not the only disturbed person in his family. His mother had a psychiatric illness known as somatization disorder. This is one of the somatoform disorders, in which affected persons present various and sundry medical-surgical complaints that are actually a product of psychiatric illness. At first glance, somatization disorder seems to have nothing in common with antisocial personality—it is in a separate diagnostic class—but the two are linked because they occur in the same families far more often than could be accounted for by coincidence. In these families, as was the case in Roger's, about 10 percent of males exhibit antisocial disorder and about 10 percent of females somatization disorder, which are excessive proportions compared to control families. This odd pairing persists through generations, so hereditary factors are presumably at work. Whether or not that proves true, the somatoform disorders, which include somatization disorder and hypochondriasis, are important in psychiatry and in medicine generally.

Somatization Disorder

Roger's mother's diagnosis is based on a history of multiple physical complaints for which no pathologic or physiologic basis is discovered. These complaints begin before age 30 and persist for several years. Females are far more likely than males to receive the diagnosis. The affected person complains about many symptoms—the diagnostic criteria call for more than 12—that generally involve several organ systems. Certain complaints are especially common in somatization disorder. These include painful menstruation, amnesia, difficulty swallowing, vaginal or rectal burning sensations, shortness of breath, double vision, arm or leg pain, and frequent vomiting. If two or three of these are present and are unexplained, they constitute a warning to doctors of possible somatization disorder. People with somatization disorder tend to describe their symptoms colorfully and with dramatic flourish, but also with a vagueness that frustrates clinicians, who try unsuccessfully to achieve greater precision by asking specific questions.

Hypochondriasis

This term denotes an overriding, unfounded concern with bodily function that persists despite reassurance. The focus tends to be on fear of specific diseases (such as cancer), and anxiety is prominent. In contrast, somatization disorder usually presents an emphasis on symptoms such as breathlessness, and anxiety is much less prominent. Indeed, persons with somatization disorder often describe their symptoms with a characteristic detached calmness that older clinicians call *la belle indifférence*.

Hypochondriasis has long posed vexing problems to medicine. For example, each year about 400,000 Americans, mostly males, have x-ray studies of their coronary arteries. Nearly all of these studies are done because of complaints of chest pain, suggesting that the heart muscle is not getting enough blood. About 100,000 of these people are found to have no coronary artery disease. Moreover, they suffer no more disease than, and they live just as long as, other people of the same age and sex. Thus their chest pain is not related to heart disease. Yet despite the encouraging result of their x-ray study, about 70,000 of these 100,000 continue to complain of chest pain and become seriously impaired vocationally and socially. Many of them have further diagnostic tests and hospitalizations. Some have surgery. Neither the discomfort and danger associated with unneeded procedures nor the enormous waste of scarce resources is warranted, because what most such people have is a treatable psychiatric illness that mimics heart disease.

Several psychiatric conditions can result in hypochondriasis. Depression is an important contributor. (Recall John's chest pain in Chapter 1.) Everything seems bleak to the depressed person, so it is understandable that minor aches may loom large and be interpreted as signs of catastrophic illness. Anxiety disorders also contribute. Anxiety's overbreathing, with its attendant numbness and tingling sensations, can produce fear of dread disease. Swallowing air is common in anxiety; the distended stomach that may result can itself be painful and it can painfully impinge on structures in the chest. Hypochondriasis is also a diagnosis in its own right in cases where depression or anxiety disorder cannot explain the complaints. Some people are apparently more aware of internal sensations than others are, and hence are likely to react with alarm and to complain about bodily twinges that the more stoic among us ignore.

Diagnosis

Historically, physicians confronted with complaints that were obscure and did not fit familiar patterns tended to make one of two possible errors. First, in the not very distant past, any unexplained set of symptoms was much too readily written off by puzzled physicians of all specialities as "hysteria" or labeled even less politely. However, careful follow-up studies of people so regarded found many of them to be suffering from a major illness such as cancer or multiple sclerosis. The symptoms wrongly explained away by the diagnosis "hysteria" were the first manifestation of these diseases. The second error has resulted in many people with somatization disorder, depression, or anxiety being subjected to needless diagnostic procedures or surgery, and often both, by doctors who either mistook a psychological problem for a physical one or were not sure what they were dealing with and fell back on the possible diagnoses that their training equipped them to confront. Most of these patients could have been treated easily and effectively if only a correct diagnosis had been made. (Physicians came to regard almost all of Roger's mother's surgery as unnecessary.)

Today both of these unhappy errors are much less likely to occur. Specific criteria have been developed that enable professionals to make a diagnosis of psychiatric illness on the basis of positive evidence. This means that a diagnosis such as hysteria cannot be used as a "wastebasket" term available for disposing of odd and mysterious symptom complexes. If positive evidence does not establish a diagnosis of psychiatric illness, the wise physician continues diagnostic studies. However, even when evidence of psychiatric illness is found, responsible physicians remember that a psychiatric diagnosis does not exclude other illnesses that may begin with vague symptoms. There is always the possibility that two disease processes are present in the same person.

Prognosis

The somatoform disorders are chronic relapsing conditions. If unnecessary medical tests and surgery can be largely avoided, they are compatible with reasonably normal life. However, flare-ups of symptoms and the consequent seeking of medical attention are likely to occur every few months. With treatment that minimizes medical attention and discourages gratuitous surgery, the prognosis becomes excellent. Successful treatment is, however, a major test of a professional's mastery of the art as well as the science of his or her craft.

Treatment

A positive diagnosis of somatoform disorder should lead to treatment and management that is likely to address effectively the concerns of the ill person. For people who suffer from hypochondriasis, specific treatments for anxiety and depression are those discussed in Chapters 1 and 5. People who, like Roger's mother, suffer from somatization disorder are best served by an ongoing relationship with a psychotherapist. Success has two key ingredients. The first is recognition by affected persons that their physical complaints tend to arise when there are problems in their lives. A perfect correspondence between life events and complaints is not always apparent, but attaining that educational objective is generally easier than is often the case in other illnesses. Second, successful therapy is based on addressing those here-and-now problems. Defining them is usually enough; solving them is a nice extra, but it is not essential to reducing symptoms. During this process, it is most important for family members (and professionals) not to back the affected person into a corner. Never say or imply that it is all in the sufferer's imagination. Leave a way out. "Sometimes pain like yours just comes and then goes away again, and doctors may never understand why." Suggestion can be very effective. "Maybe that will happen to you." In this way crises can be managed in a couple of visits, which can be repeated as often as necessary. Most often such visits are infrequent.

Chapter

9

Sex, Syphilis, and AIDS

□ □ □

AMONG the larger creatures of our planet, humans are the undisputed champions when it comes to interest in sex and in the performance of sexual activities. Nearly all animals are periodic, often seasonal, in sexual interest; with them, sex serves the purpose of procreation only. Primates are exceptions: Their sexual activity serves to create and strengthen social bonding. And humans are the most exceptional of all. With us, sexual interest can be high at any time for both males and females. A very large proportion of our energy and time is devoted to sex. We prolong the act of copulation itself much longer than any other mammal, and we perform it more often. Not to mention the time spent flirting, preening, seeking a partner, and in sexual foreplay, as well as the attention lavished on sex in our music, humor, and conversation. And during much of the time when we are not directly occupied with sex, we are preoccupied with it. No other animal is even in the same league.

Little wonder that sex is at the root of many problems of concern to psychiatry. These problems have three basic themes. (1) Our sexual behavior, like any other behavior, is subject to dis-ease. (2) Sexually transmitted diseases have helped form our society. Many species of disease-causing microorganisms have adapted over evolutionary time to exploit human sexuality by becoming sexually transmitted. Those that have succeeded have forced society to respond in ways that have contributed to the definition of aberrant sexual behaviors and to the imposition of sanctions against them. As was the case with drug abuse, these definitions have varied with the perceived risk of personal and social incapacity that is associated with particular behaviors. In past eras these reactions have been mainly to syphilis; today they are mainly to AIDS. These diseases have led us not only to alter profoundly specific sexual behaviors and attitudes but also to intense conflicts about the meaning and nature of sexual behavior, and about the balance between individual rights and the common good. (3) Finally, syphilis and AIDS directly and profoundly involve brain tissue and hence psychiatric medicine.

Syphilis

Syphilis destroyed European innocence. The disease appeared in Europe about 1493; perhaps Columbus' sailors actually did bring it back from the New World. But whatever its source, syphilis swept across the continent and from there throughout the world in the ensuing centuries. Any organ of the body could be affected, so an ill person often had a bewildering pattern of signs and symptoms. Syphilis was known as the great imitator, because it had to be considered a possible diagnosis given almost any combination of signs and symptoms. This included psychiatric signs and symptoms: Nearly half of the cases of tertiary syphilis (the most advanced stage of the disease) produced brain disease only. Recognition of this did not come easily. The logical and scientific struggle occasioned by syphilis produced a sea change in concepts of brain disease, behavior, and the relationship between them. This history is outlined in Box 7.

Box 7   Syphilis and General Parasis of the Insane

General parasis of the insane, or GPI, is the major brain disorder caused by syphilis. The disease features a personality change—often depression but sometimes mania or paranoia—that, untreated, is followed quickly by gross intellectual deficits and death within several months to a year or two. By the end of the Napoleonic wars in the early nineteenth century, GPI was an epidemic disease in Europe and had spread to North America. It was regarded as a distinct illness, and most authorities thought it was caused by excessive use of alcohol and by the lifestyle of the lower social classes. However, the lower social classes also had an excess of syphilis, and slowly the association between GPI and syphilis became recognized. Establishing that GPI was in fact a manifestation of syphilis caused bitter controversies. Even the Wasserman test, developed early in this century, which made the diagnosis of syphilitic infection secure, did not settle the matter though in retrospect, the evidence seems overwhelming: Within the limits of laboratory error, every person with GPI had a positive Wasserman test—had syphilis. However, even when faced with that evidence, many authorities simply could not accept the idea that an infection could affect personality in such a specific way. Hereditary "taint," alcoholism, mental strain, spiritual lapses, sexual excess—all continued to have their influential champions as alternative causes.

It was only through the actual demonstration of spirochetes in the brain tissue of all persons with GPI, and in no persons without GPI, that the matter was settled. This was the first demonstration that a specific brain disease resulting from a specific cause could be recognized through a specific behavioral syndrome. Moreover, the evidence was so conclusive that ever since, researchers have attempted to reach the same standard with other major brain diseases—and have never yet succeeded.

Persons affected by syphilitic brain disease displayed the range of behavioral pathology described in all the preceding chapters. Most often a subtle change of personality in the direction of decreasing intellectual and social efficiency was the first evidence of disease. This was frequently masked by a grandiose, manic-like state or paranoia. Usually within a year of the first signs of brain disease, however, dementia came to dominate.

In the 1920s, about 30 percent of severe mental illness was attributed to syphilis. Until the development of penicillin in the late 1940s, its effect on the brain made syphilis by far the largest single contributor to the populations of mental hospitals. Syphilis in all of its manifestations had become an extremely common disease. Among prostitutes in the United States, the rate of infection was 50 percent or higher. Among young American men examined for the draft during World War I, 13 percent had syphilis or gonorrhea or both. It also affected newborn children, sentencing them to profound mental and physical disability and often to death. It was feared as few diseases before or since—until AIDS.

Syphilis is caused by a spirochete, a form of bacteria. Soon after its first appearance in Europe, the disease became known to be sexually transmitted, and to be transmitted from mothers to their unborn children. It also soon became known that one's chances of contracting the disease were increased by having numbers of sexual partners. By relaxing inhibitions, alcohol increased the risk of sexual contact and syphilitic infection. Thus, syphilis became associated with deviation from strict monogamy, alcoholic excesses, and an undisciplined lifestyle. Some segments of society viewed syphilis as a deserved punishment. The socially imposed restrictions on sexual activity outside of marriage known (unfairly) as Victorian morality followed. This change in behavior, the "safe sex" of that day, partly contained the epidemic.

Syphilis affected sexual attitudes and behaviors in other ways both large and small. For example, only about 5 percent of U.S.males were circumcised until early in this century, when it became widely believed that circumcision protected a man against sexually trans-mitted disease (The evidence is inconclusive.) Then the rate went rapidly up to 90 percent.

Syphilis was also the subject of a scientific effort that greatly advanced our knowledge of biology. Scientific investigation of this

disease contributed significantly to our present sophisticated ap-
preciation of the relationships between pathogenic microorganisms
and their hosts, which are extremely complex and interwoven over a
long history. An agent that causes disease, a pathogen, is effective
until its hosts have evolved defensive measures. Then the pathogen
must respond, usually by a genetic change that defeats the host's new
defenses, forcing a further adaptation if the host is to survive. And so
on. This evolutionary process has gone on for so long that most
pathogens target one animal species and do not infect others or, if
they do infect others, do not produce disease. Humans share in this
animal background. But humans have greatly augmented the ancient
weaponry by adding to it behavioral change and scientific biology.

Since about 1945, our "safe sex" defenses against syphilis have
been largely superseded by scientific ones. Our current main defense
is scientific knowledge—our understanding of how to produce and
use antibiotics. One social side effect of successful antibiotic treatment of syphilis (with help from the birth control pill) was the
"sexual revolution" proclaimed during 1960s which, in fact, is perhaps more accurately regarded as a return to pre-syphilis sexual
behavior. However, syphilis remains a latent threat. As the history of
disease emphatically tells us, syphilis could develop resistance to our
antibiotics and overwhelm them. New cases of syphilis have been
increasing and a large reservoir of infected persons are available to
transmit the disease. Indeed, in America today, slightly more new
cases of syphilis are reported each year than new cases of AIDS. The
difference is that, at least for now, syphilis can be effectively treated.

AIDS

In the United States, AIDS first reached epidemic proportions among
homosexual males. Why this group was especially vulnerable is still
not clear, but as with syphilis, one factor is the large number of sexual
contacts among them. Most affected homosexual males were extremely active sexually. In response to AIDS, homosexuals responded
much as heterosexuals did to syphilis—by embracing monogamy and
"safe sex." The rate at which new cases are reported is still rising, but

it has recently slowed and may begin to decline. For years to come, however, the homosexual population will be ravaged by one of the cruelest of diseases.

From homosexuals, the disease has spread to intravenous drug users, who are now the major focus of the epidemic. They in turn are spreading the disease to their sexual partners, usually women, who transmit it to about 30 percent of the children they bear. Hospitals serving poor areas are reporting that about 1 in 50 newborns carries the disease. Transmission from female to male through sexual activity does occur, but it is uncommon among North American and European populations. In Africa, however, the sexes are affected with equal frequency. Some experts think that this is a result of the greater incidence in Africa of other sexually transmitted diseases, which produce genital sores that may increase susceptibility to AIDS. Other experts see the African situation as a deadly warning of what Western societies can expect.

AIDS is having an effect on sexual behavior similar to that of syphilis before it. The brief respite from Victorian morality that penicillin and new methods of birth control bought us has been interrupted if not ended entirely. There is excellent reason for this. In 1989, AIDS was the eleventh leading cause of death in the USA. By 1991 it was in eighth place, tied with suicide.

Like syphilis, AIDS can affect all organ systems. Current evidence suggests that it always affects the brain, whereas syphilis spares the brain in about 50 percent of cases. The brain disease of AIDS may be mild, but in about 60 percent of cases it is severe, although the primary results of brain tissue involvement can be hard to separate from the secondary results of infections and tumors that AIDS produces in other organs.

AIDS brain disease is nearly always manifested in a dementing process. Malaise, loss of interest, and mental slowing appear first. These signs and symptoms are followed by patchy loss of recent memory, difficulty concentrating, and disordered progression of thought. Mood disorder or paranoia may create diagnostic problems in the early stages, but intellectual defects soon predominate.

AIDS has been concentrated among male homosexuals, a predominantly literate group that knows it is at high risk. As a result, doctors are often asked to order diagnostic tests for persons who are not ill but live in constant fear of the disease. Such requests are easy to understand, and usually a test is warranted. But a significant proportion of such people are not reassured by a negative test and request that it be repeated, often several times. Again, there is logic underlying the request. The length of the interval between infection and the development of bodily changes that make testing reliable is not precisely known: It may be several months to years. Add to that uncertainty the anxiety, depression, and fearfulness that can be pervasive enough to suggest a personality change consistent with early AIDS, and a sad human problem emerges.

Reminiscent of syphilis, AIDS is today the impetus behind another massive research effort, and, as in the early efforts to combat syphilis, solutions appear to be beyond our grasp. But our species's history suggests that AIDS too will be repulsed by medicine, though probably not defeated completely. It will surely remain a latent threat.

Meanwhile, the research is yielding fascinating information. AIDS is caused by a retrovirus, an organism that was studied little before the AIDS epidemic. Now retroviruses are regarded as one of the most promising vehicles for introducing corrective genes into our cells as treatment for genetic disease. In nature, they have been doing that for millennia. Some of our genes—estimates range from 1 percent to 10 percent—were bequeathed by retroviruses that attacked our ancestors: Our evolutionary forebearers took over the invading genes and adapted them to their own purposes.

Homosexuality

Homosexuality is not today considered as a psychiatric illness in the United States. However, there are two reasons why it should be discussed here. First, homosexual behavior was once an official diagnosis in America, and many still regard it as a behavioral aberration. Mental health professionals get a steady stream of inquiries about it from individuals concerned about their own sexuality and from families who have a homosexual member. Also, in much of the world, homosexuality remains a diagnosable condition. Second, and more important to psychiatry today, male homosexuality has been central to the spread of AIDS.

The proportion of the adult male population whose sexual orientation is more or less exclusively homosexual is not known with any precision, but 3 percent to 4 percent would be a reasonable estimate. Even less is known about the proportion of female homosexuals (lesbians), but it is probably much smaller.

Some male homosexuals are effeminate as children. As adolescents, as many as 80 percent become aware that they are sexually attracted to persons of their own sex and indifferent to the opposite sex. Others develop homosexual feelings later in life, sometimes after marrying and having children. One possible explanation of some apparently late-onset homosexuality is that in America, acknowledgement, perhaps even recognition of homosexual inclinations, can be long delayed because of strong cultural sanctions against it.

Sexual activity among homosexuals varies. Anal intercourse is common among males. Some gays are always the receptive partner, some always the active one, others play both roles at different times. Fellatio is frequently practiced. However, the transmission of sexual disease among homosexual males has taken place mainly within a particular group: members of the bathhouse subculture. These men's sexual behavior was distinguished by its anonymity and promiscuity, and each individual's sexual contact with sometimes hundreds of men—mostly strangers and over a short time—created an ideal environment for the proliferation of sexually transmitted diseases of all sorts.

Bathhouse culture was unique. A participant would rent a private cubicles and, when he sought sexual contact, would leave the door open so that passing men could look in. Sometimes hints of the sort of sexual activity desired were displayed—a lubricant for anal intercourse, for example. An interested man would stop at the door and, if attracted, ask to come in, sometimes only with a questioning look. Agreement was signaled by a nod and the door was closed. We can use the past tense in describing bathhouses because those facilities and the sexual behaviors they promoted have been largely eliminated in response to the AIDS epidemic.

Other homosexuals form more or less monogamous relationships; many couples live together for years. Descriptions of these relationships make it clear that real affectional ties develop in a pattern entirely analogous to heterosexual marriage. The incidence of AIDS is only marginally higher in this group than among the general population.

Lesbian sexual behavior tends strongly toward subtle, less overtly genital behavior than that of male homosexuals. Women also tend to have a much smaller number of sexual partners. AIDS has not emerged as a problem in this group.

■ *If You Are Concerned About Homosexuality*

We do not choose to become homosexual or heterosexual. That choice is made for us by biologic and social mechanisms that are not yet understood. Not homosexuals, their parents, or society at large causes the condition. Being dressed or otherwise treated as a member of the wrong physical sex does not produce homosexuality. Neither psychiatry nor any other profession or putative profession has a treatment that will change sexual orientation. Of course, the availability of effective treatment is not a test for the presence or absence of disease. More telling is the fact that homosexuality per se creates no dis-ease to be treated. If homosexuality is simply accepted as a fact of life, it is perfectly compatible with a happy life, social productivity, and stable relationships.

Problems do arise because of the rejection of homosexuality by much of society and the resulting tendency of some homosexuals themselves to reject their sexuality. This has not always been the case. From the classical world through the Renaissance, homosexuality appears to have been accepted and regarded as within the range of normal behavior. For whatever reason, that acceptance was partly withdrawn in the nineteenth century. Restoration of it seemed well underway, but progress has been interrupted by the AIDS epidemic. This setback is especially tragic because it is acceptance that homosexuals need—acceptance by themselves, by their families, and by society at large.

Transsexualism

Transsexuals believe they inhabit the body of the wrong sex, which is probably why they are often sent to psychiatrists. Transsexuals acknowledge their physical sex, which is most often male, as a biologic fact. But they nevertheless insist that somehow a mistake was made—

that their instincts, minds, and "true sex" are actually those of the opposite sex. By age 3 or 4, biologically male transsexuals may try to dress in "girls" clothing, give themselves feminine names, and prefer to play with girls (by whom, surprisingly, they are nearly always accepted and welcomed). Transsexuals are homosexual. They differ from other homosexuals in that they come to physicians seeking surgery and hormone treatments to correct what they regard as an error of nature. No known treatment can alter their conviction that their biologic sex is incorrect.

Over the past few decades, surgical techniques have been developed to the extent that sex change has become a practical possibility for both men and women. Surgery is used to fashion substitute sex organs and to remove breasts from women. Males have their external genitalia removed and artificial vaginas constructed. Hormones produce further changes. The surgery has become technically quite satisfactory. The artificial sex organs are reported to work well, even to the point of enabling the postoperative patient to experience orgasm and making it possible to deceive long term sexual partners. However, there is little agreement about the overall effectiveness of surgery in helping people achieve a satisfying life. In order to establish a valid prognosis, there must be further long-term study comparing transsexuals who have had the surgery to those who have not.

Paraphilias

Paraphilias are characterized by unusual or bizarre behaviors engaged in for attaining sexual excitement. Most of these behaviors are rare or inconsequential. I shall describe only the most common and most distressing to the public at large. Paraphiliacs themselves do not regard themselves as ill; they have no dis-ease. However, they realize that most of society considers them deviant.

Transvestism is the practice of dressing in the clothing of the opposite sex in order to achieve sexual arousal. Sometimes the costuming is a complete outfit. More often single articles (underwear, for example) are involved. In this case the behavior constitutes a *fetish*.

Usually there is a ritual involving the articles of clothing and the manner of wearing them. The sexual arousal usually precedes masturbation or, less often, sexual intercourse. Almost all transvestites are male heterosexuals. None seek sex-change operations. Few are dangerous or in any way disabled. Unless some associated behavior such as stealing clothing from neighborhood clotheslines makes them a public nuisance, their behavior amounts to an harmless quirk. A strange quirk to most of us, but only a quirk.

Pedophilia is a sexual preference for prepubertal children. Child molestation is an abhorred crime that is surprisingly common: As many as 25 percent of female and 10 percent of male children are affected. Some 30 percent to 35 percent of arrested sex offenders are pedophiliacs; nearly all are male, and nearly all knew the victim as a relative or neighborhood child. The onset of pedophilia may occur at any age, but most often it is in mid-life. Rarely is significant physical injury done. The assault is on the emotional well-being of the child.

Although several experimental treatment programs based mainly based on behavior modification are being tested on pedophiliacs, none has yet proved effective in preventing repeat offenses. For those who must comfort or treat victims, a few guidelines may be useful. Remain calm and matter-of-fact in front of the child. Prosecute the offender, safeguard the child, and express outrage—but not in front of the child. Most often the child has not been physically injured and has been seduced rather than forced. An adult's expression of emotional revulsion may induce unwarranted feelings of guilt in the child. Worse, the reactions of adults may exacerbate the damage done to the child. Children victimized by a pedophiliac will not forget, but they will slowly integrate the experience in a much healthier way if it is *not* complicated by memories of emotionally aroused, condemning adults.

Exhibitionism is the display of genitalia to an unsuspecting stranger. The exhibitionist is male; he usually displays an erect penis. Victims are female. The exhibitionist is generally most rewarded by screams or signs of fright in his victim; he seeks to startle and so to dominate. Lack of response is a defeat. Exhibitionists are rarely aggressive apart from the exposure itself, and there is little physical danger. However, there is a hidden danger for the victim. Many women report that along with being startled and feeling revulsion, they also experienced sexual arousal. This seems so perverse that many women are ashamed, keep it secret, and worry a great deal about it. No need. It is a normal reaction of many women, best simply acknowledged and forgotten.

Heterosexual Adjustment

Perhaps anxiety about sex has always been a problem for adolescents and young adults, but it appears that many of us suffer from uncertainty about our sexual "adequacy" in later years as well. Over the past few decades, sexuality has been studied intensively by mental health professionals, and treatments for sexual dis-ease have been developed, refined, and made widely available. The disorders have been defined as follows, but critical revisions are under way.

• *Sexual desire disorders* Otherwise known as "low sex drive," these conditions may affect up to 20 percent of the population. However, agreement on what is "normal" in this context has not yet been reached. In practice, this condition usually means that one member of a sexual pair has less desire for sexual contact than the other.

• *Sexual arousal disorders* This designation applies to erectile failure in males either before or during sexual activity, to inadequate vaginal lubrication in women, or to lack of subjective pleasure in either males or females. Medications, including especially those used to treat high blood pressure and those useful in psychiatric diseases, are frequent causes of erectile failure. Vaginal lubrication requires normal hormonal status coupled with adequate sexual arousal. Psychological factors and misinformation are common causes of arousal disorders in both sexes.

• *Orgasm disorders* In women, this is known as "inhibited female orgasm." Up to 20 percent of normal women may never experience orgasm. The reasons are unknown in most cases. Premature ejaculation and delayed ejaculation in males, are both grouped here. Male disorders show a definite age effect; young males tend to be premature, older ones delayed.

Young males can usually learn control, but the best approach to delayed ejaculation appears to be to accept it as a normal aspect of aging.

• *Sexual pain disorder* Pain upon intercourse in women may result from inadequate vaginal lubrication or from normal sexual activity after a period of abstinence. In both sexes, but especially in females, infection is a common cause.

Efforts to agree on diagnostic criteria and to develop treatments for these disorders have been constructive and have been rewarded with considerable success. Anyone affected by one of these disorders is well advised to see a qualified professional. However, charlatans abound. Before entering a treatment program, get recommendations from local professional associations.

6

THE FUTURE OF PSYCHIATRY

∎∎∎

To SUCCESSFULLY treat disease, we must understand it. That is the ongoing task of all of medicine, including psychiatry. The great recent advances in understanding psychiatric illness are an outgrowth of two complementary processes. First, a great deal of underbrush had to be cleared away before testable hypotheses based on the evolving biologic sciences could be developed. The nature of the underbrush and the process by which the clearing is proceeding— though far along it is not yet complete—will be a continuing theme of this chapter. Second, it had to be demonstrated that the methods of the biologic sciences could be applied to the study of behavior and its disorders. Studies of families (especially studies of adopted children and twins) strongly supported genetic transmission, and this, coupled with the success of pharmacologic treatments, convinced a cadre of professionals that there was a biology of mental illness, and that it was accessible to scientific study. They staked their careers on those convictions and they are winning big.

The following chapter gives an overview of developing brain science and a preview of its probable impact on those affected by mental illness. Because the focus here is on the future, there may seem to be little benefit for persons like George and Jerry whose illnesses we described in earlier chapters. However, advances in the brain sciences are occurring at an unprecedented rate. There is an excellent chance that those who are now ill will benefit significantly. For the more distant future, we should be thinking about preventing mental disease altogether.

Chapter

10

The Causes of Mental Illness
□ □ □

TODAY, two inarguable assertions can be made about every disease and condition described in this book: Genes contribute to causing each of them, and environments contribute to causing each of them. For several decades there seemed to be an irreconcilable contradiction between those statements, and theories on the cause of psychiatric illness tended toward extreme polarization—nature versus nurture. The apparent contradiction is now being reconciled in a way that is yielding previews of psychiatry's future: Not nature alone, and not nurture alone; both are necessary links in the causal chain leading to disease. This formulation implies radically different research methods that are now coming on line, and in the longer term, it implies radically different treatments and preventive measures aimed at the mental illnesses. And it promises to raise radically provocative questions for our society.

The Indictment of Genes

It has long been known that relatives of people affected with any psychiatric illness are more likely to develop that same illness than are members of the general population. For close relatives, the risk for most important diseases is increased 10 to 20 times. More recently, evidence has established that except for psychiatric illness caused by infections, such as syphilis, this relationship owes much more to inherited genes than to family environment. People adopted as infants and reared in average families develop the illnesses of their biologic parents, not those of their adoptive parents. In fact, children develop the illnesses of their biologic parents at virtually identical rates whether they are reared with those parents or are adopted as infants into non-related families usually screened by adoption agencies for psychiatric health. Especially notable are studies of children of normal parents adopted into homes wherein an adoptive parent develops a psychiatric illness. These children do not have a higher-than-average risk for the illness of the adoptive parent or for any other illness.

Other studies have shown that identical twins, who possess identical genes, are much more likely to share the same illness—to be *concordant*—than are fraternal twins, who share only 50 percent of their genes. The identical twin of a person with a mental illness runs between a 20 percent and a 50 percent risk of having the same illness. Equivalent percentages for fraternal twins, who share only 50 percent of their genes, are significantly smaller. These results have been amplified by studies of identical twins reared apart, from infancy, in separate adoptive homes. Such twins are strikingly alike in mental health regardless of the conditions of their rearing.

Recognition of the importance of genes in psychiatric disease represents an about-face from the view that prevailed a couple of decades ago, but it is based on solid evidence. Enough studies have been done on enough diseases, and on enough strategic populations of twins reared together and apart, and on enough adopted persons and their biologic and adoptive relatives, to secure a place for genes in the causation of nearly all the psychiatric illnesses discussed in this book. The evidence is widely regarded as conclusive by behavior scientists.

The Indictment of Environment

Twin studies also provide the clearest evidence that environment too makes an essential contribution to disease. Though identical pairs are more likely than members of the general population to share the same illnesses, they do not always do so. It is clear from the concordance estimates we have cited that between 50 and 80 percent of identical pairs do not share the same illness; they are *discordant*. Because identical twins have identical genes at conception, any differences between them must have originated after conception—that is, broadly speaking, they must be environmental in origin. *Environmental* in this sense includes more than social milieu. It also comprises all non-genetic events, including, as will be seen, the rearrangement and inactivation of genes themselves, aspects of which appears to be random in critical respects. Luck may turn out to be an underestimated contributor to outcome that will have to be added to nature and nurture.

A proportion of those discordant twins are not entirely free of illness; indeed, many seem to have lesser forms of the conditions that affect their co-twins. For example, cyclothymic mood swings (which fall well short of mania and major depression, as described in Chapter 2) occur in about 15 percent of identical twins of people who have bipolar illness. Schizoid disorders (which resemble schizophrenia but are less severe) occur in about 20 percent of twins of schizophrenics. Such twins probably possess the genetic fault associated with the illness, but a relatively advantageous post-conception course led to its lesser severity. Events occurring after conception must also account for the many differences in severity of illness between twins who are concordant for illness. For example, when identical cotwins develop schizophrenia, their ages at onset of the illness, a good estimator of severity, are on average 5 years apart.

Even more telling evidence for the role of environment in mental illness is that in any twin study, some identical twins of affected persons remain absolutely normal, free of any hint of illness. Moreover, in the case of at least one illness, schizophrenia, the children of discordant identical pairs provide important confirmatory evidence. Children of the normal member of a discordant pair are just as likely to develop schizophrenia as are children of the ill member.

Because the normal twins must have possessed the faulty genetic material in order to transmit it, we can be certain that having pathologic genes is not sufficient to cause illness. Gene carriers may escape schizophrenia entirely—though some of their children may not.

Gene-Environment Interaction

Given the facts that emerged from twin and family studies, many behavior scientists adopted a theoretical formulation called *gene-environment interaction* to slip between the horns of the nature-nurture dilemma. In this view, genes predispose one to—that is, increase the probability of one's contracting—disease, but they do not absolutely determine it. On the other hand, without the predisposing genes, developing the disease is most unlikely, perhaps even impossible.

If the genes must be faulty in order for disease to develop, what contribution does environment make? Adoption and twin studies strongly suggest that the environmental conditions involved are not extreme ones. In the adoption studies, for example, the environments were effectively random; thus there is no reason to believe that the environments of adopted children who developed a disease differed in any systematic way from the environments of adopted children who did not develop a disease. It has been even more difficult to find systematic environmental differences that could explain why identical twins or other biologic siblings reared with their biologic parents often have different outcomes: One might develop a major disease while another remained entirely well despite being reared in a similar environment. The explanation is probably that the environmental factors predisposing to disease are not spectacular aberrations. For people possessing normal genes, they would be routine features of everyday life. But these same features may greatly harm persons with faulty genes.

The theory of gene-environment interaction worked to everyone's satisfaction so long as both "gene" and "environment" were abstractions and there was no need to specify exactly what one meant when one used either term. But no longer. Scientists are increasingly able to specify and measure the physical and chemical properties of genes. And that ability is changing the world. As part of this process, some connotations of the word *gene* itself have become obsolete; it has been replaced by terms such as *DNA segment* in formal scientific communication. More important, our growing understanding of the physical chemistry of DNA, the constituent of genes, is leaving environmental studies far behind. This imbalance has profound implications for medicine and society. To grapple with these implications, it is important first to clear away debris left over from past popular misunderstandings of biology. One especially misleading assumption has been that, at conception, an individual's genetic make-up and all gene activity are set and determined for the rest of life and that nothing can be done about genetic disease. To understand the scope and tools of modern biologic psychiatry, it is necessary to know that assumption is not valid. The following brief overview of modern genetics is a first step in that direction.

▪ From DNA to Disease ▪

We inherit DNA, deoxyribonucleic acid, from our parents. DNA contains, in the form of the genetic code, the information needed for life. The coding components of DNA are four relatively small molecules—the nucleic acids—linked together in such a way as to form long chains. Our chains of DNA are separated into packages, the chromosomes. Normally there are 46 chromosomes in each of our cells, 23 from our mother, and 23 from our father. The order in which the four nucleic acids line up in the DNA chains within each chromosome is inherited from the parent who gave us that chromosome: It follows that half our DNA is arranged in sequences transmitted from our mothers, half from our fathers. With exceptions unimportant for our purposes, each cell of our body contains about 6 billion nucleic acids.

DNA is the stuff of life. It can make exact copies of itself, thereby making reproduction possible. DNA also has two basic functions pertinent to psychiatric disease. First, the order of nucleic acids in DNA determines the structure of our proteins—the bricks, mortar, and tools of our physical selves. Second, DNA helps regulate the amount of protein produced at any given moment throughout life. Together, differences in protein structure and differences in amounts of protein produced account for all the biologic diversity among us. This diversity includes predisposition to disease.

■■■

The Structure of Proteins

Some DNA segments code for specific amino acids to be linked together to form proteins. The four coding nucleic acids are adenine, cytosine, guanine, and thymine. A sequence of three nucleic acids codes for one amino acid out of the 20 that make up our proteins. For example, if we let the initials A, C, G, and T stand for the four nucleic acids, A-C-G codes for the amino acid threonine, T-T-T for phenylalanine, and so on. When decoded, a segment of DNA some several thousand nucleic acids long contains the information needed to make one chain of amino acids. Such a chain of amino acids may itself constitute a complete protein, but most chains are processed after their constituent amino acids are linked together—to form, for example, together with other chains, a more complex protein.

DNA supplies the information of life; proteins organize and perform its work. It helps to think of two types of proteins. *Structural proteins* make up the structure of our bodies. They are the materials of which our cells, the matrix of our bones, and the solids in our blood are composed. They manufacture our non-protein molecules, such as hormones and neurotransmitters. Structural proteins incorporate for use or transport small molecules such as minerals, fats, sugars, and vitamins. *Regulatory proteins*, on the other hand, increase or decrease the production of structural proteins by attaching to specific DNA segments: Such unions instruct DNA segments to increase or decrease production.

Through a chance event—a *mutation*—one nucleic acid may be substituted for another. For example, in one type of mutation, C may replace the second G in G-G-C, making G-C-C; then the amino acid alanine is substituted for glycine in the protein coded for by that DNA segment. If a mutation occurs in the DNA of a germ cell (egg or sperm), it can be passed on from generation to generation. Mutations are basically chance events; they occur at random. What effect a mutation has depends on where it happens to occur.

A difference in DNA structure that results from mutation may be entirely without practical effect on life; or it may alter a protein product just enough to make it slightly less efficient or slightly more efficient; or it may alter a protein product enough to predispose to disease. In our example, the substitution of alanine for glycine in a specific protein is associated with the disease phenylketonuria, a major illness that may cause profound mental retardation. The affected protein normally breaks down another amino acid, phenylalanine. But because of the substitution, this process is ineffective, leading to poisoning with by-products of phenylalanine's faulty digestion. As is typical of what we are learning about the complexity of diseases, 22 other alterations in the same protein, caused by different mutations, are now known. It is important to note that the effective treatment is an adjustment of environment, the elimination of phenylalanine from the diet. Without the environmental co-determinant, there is no disease.

The Regulation of Protein Production

We respond to environmental challenges through DNA's second major function, regulation of protein production. The response can be instantaneous or occur years after the challenge. DNA responds to its environment by acting in conjunction with other molecules to control the amounts of structural protein produced. Regulatory proteins are one essential class of such molecules, but non-protein molecules which attach at specially configured DNA sites, can decrease or increase the production of particular proteins and there are additional levels of regulation not directly involving DNA. The effects of these mechanisms are finely graded across a range from complete blocking of production to massive increases. Like structural sites, regulatory sites on DNA are also subject to mutation and consequently to changes in functional capacity.

The substances that unite with DNA or regulate at other levels are themselves the direct or indirect products of DNA segments. Some may be produced in response to housekeeping demands, such as those imposed by internal timing mechanisms or "clocks". But the production of regulatory molecules is also our response to changes in our external environment: DNA enables us to mount finely modulated responses to ongoing changes in our external world. Box 8 illustrates gene-environment interaction through the "stress" protein or "heat shock" system.

DNA Change and Disease

Inheritance is not rigid, unchanging, or unforgiving. We have emphasized that DNA segments actively respond to moment-to-moment changes in environment throughout life. Moreover, although the structure of DNA—and therefore the structures of proteins produced in response to specific environments—is largely determined at conception, there are exceptions that will probably turn out to be important to psychiatric illness. DNA itself changes. DNA segments involved with immune responses, and those whose functions are less well known, rearrange themselves throughout life, changing location on the same chromosome or even moving to a different chromosome. Such changes can have important regulatory consequences.

Other DNA segments are inactivated, apparently at random, very early in the development of an embryo. This occurs when paired DNA segments, one from the father, the other from the mother, would produce too much protein if both were decoded. Evolution's answer was to develop machinery to inactivate one segment, leaving its paired mate to produce protein throughout life. Even though other genes presumably initiate the inactivation, it is thought that random processes (luck) determine which DNA segments, maternal or paternal, are inactivated in each cell of the embryo. Because there are few cells at that stage in development, and because the inactivation is passed on to all of their progeny cells, it becomes possible by chance to inactivate significantly more maternal than paternal DNA, or vice versa. The resulting mix of protein product may be advantageous, neutral, or disadvantageous to the organism. Some diseases are manifest because the disproportionate inactivation of DNA coding for a normal functioning protein, has left its abnormal partner to manage by itself, however ineffectually. Here again, sheer chance probably plays a significant role. (The philosophically inclined may note that determinism is being undone by one of the sciences that helped give rise to it.)

DNA, Environment, and Diseases

Direct studies of human DNA became feasible just a few years ago. Perhaps 1978, the year in which comprehensive mapping of human DNA was first seen as a remote possibility, is a good year to mark as the beginning of an era destined to change radically our world, our understanding of mental illness, and our view of ourselves.

The first step in successful searches for the causes of genetic disease has been to locate approximately the site of a disease-associated DNA segment on a specific chromosome. Then the location of that DNA segment is pinpointed by locating markers on either side of it. The next step is determining the segment's nucleic acid sequence. Then, working from the genetic code, it is possible to infer the structure of any protein produced by the segment. This is a laborious process but it has been reached by research into some human diseases.

The next steps have not yet been successfully mounted, and especially if all or part of the DNA segment is regulatory, how to proceed is not so evident. Considerable trial-and-error research may be needed, but active workers in the field have no doubt that the technology now in hand will enable us to define the mechanisms through which regulation is accomplished. This entails learning to what environmental factors a specific regulatory mechanism responds, what protein product or products it regulates, and whether it increases or decreases production of those products in response to a given change in the environment. Next, DNA segments associated with disease, the equivalent normal DNA segments, and the protein products of each will be directly compared to define precisely the differences between them. Finally, treatments will be sought that bypass or neutralize damage done by the defective segment. Incredibly, modern research suggests that for some diseases, it may be possible actually to replace or repair the faulty DNA itself.

Investigation of disease through molecular genetics is just one aspect of a vast revolution now gaining momentum. This revolution promises to have an impact on human life more profound even than that of computers or atomic power. The U.S. National Institutes of Health has announced a target date of 2002 for completion of a map of human DNA. In fact, the map will probably be finished before that

Box 8   Heat Shock Proteins

An example of this finely tuned relationship between DNA and environment is provided by the so-called "heat shock" proteins, often called "stress proteins." They are produced by cells subject to one of several aversive stimuli-heat, which explains the historical origin of the name, but also certain drugs, lack of oxygen, hydrogen peroxide, infections, and hormones, among others. Affected cells immediately slow or stop production of proteins appropriate under normal conditions and then augment production by up to 100-fold of small heat shock proteins. Some of these small proteins are known to be regulatory and to combine directly with DNA. One effect of heat shock proteins is to shut down routine operations, thus protecting cellular machinery. Another effect is to mark the place on DNA where routine decoding was stopped, in order to facilitate prompt restarting when conditions again become favorable. Production of heat shock proteins and cessation of normal cell metabolism persist for variable periods. Once induced, subsequent aversive stimuli cause their production to increase over previous levels. There is a hint here of "memory" for stressful events.

date, because the United States is not acting alone—all scientifically advanced nations are participating in one way or another—and because advances in technique are coming at a prodigious rate. Maps of other organisms are also being developed: some faster than the human map, most slower, but all inexorably.

With progress in mapping is coming the ability to manipulate the structure of DNA. The implications are awesome. We are rapidly gaining knowledge and control that will make possible manipulation of our world's biology with no intrinsic physical limits to that power now apparent. It is entirely possible that through genetic manipula-

There is a general lesson in the evolution of heat shock that will be returned to in connection with brain proteins. DNA segments coding for heat shock proteins have nearly the same structure in organisms from bacteria to man. Biologists describe them as "highly conserved through evolution" which means that since few mutations have been tolerated, the products must be essential to life. While the structure of heat shock proteins is similar in all organisms, the conditions which initiate their production—their regulation—has changed dramatically over evolutionary time. For example, the cells of humans, arctic fishes, and soybeans produce proteins of nearly the same structure in response to heat. But human cells respond at about 100 degrees Fahrenheit, fish cells at about 10 degrees, and soybean cells when the summer sun becomes hot. Evolution has conserved DNA coding for heat shock proteins, but it has changed DNA coding for regulation of production so that the condition responded to is appropriate to environmental demands on the three different organisms.

tions, we may become able to prevent virtually all disease; increase, say, our offspring's intelligence or musical ability; make crops and farm animals more productive; and even design new organisms that are as complex as any now known, including ourselves. Such prospects are beyond our present technical ability, but not so far as to be out of the question. This emerging knowledge cannot be left for scientists and physicians alone to understand and use. A truly informed and empowered citizenry will be needed to make wise decisions about the opportunities and dangers of the biologic revolution. If we are to cope sensibly with this new world of biology, an immense educational effort lies ahead.

The New Genetics and the New Psychiatry

How do we get from our present psychiatry to the "promised land" of molecular biology? And what will happen when we do? Molecular genetic research in psychiatry is following the same strategy as in general medicine: Isolate DNA segments associated with pathologic behaviors, determine their nucleic acid sequence, and infer from that sequence the amino acid structure of any protein product and how its production is regulated, comparing normal with abnormal at each step. So far, several brain diseases (including rarer psychiatric diseases) have been linked to specific chromosomes. However, among the common psychiatric disorders, only the linkage of Alzheimer's disease to chromosome 21 and that of bipolar illness to the X chromosome can be considered reasonably certain; and even in these instances only a small proportion of families with affected members exhibit those linkages. This is to be expected; experience with genetic disease suggests that most common diseases are associated with more than one distinct genetic mechanism—and often with several. The tools we need are available, and the mapping of diseases will be refined and repeated in the coming years until conclusions become certain.

So we must think ahead to a day soon to come when we will be comparing behaviorly normal and abnormal DNA segments in test tubes. When such comparison becomes possible, investigation of psychiatric disease will face a stumbling block that, though far from unique to psychiatry, does underscore past lapses of behavior science. We have effectively no knowledge of the environments that interact with DNA to yield disease. We cannot expect to understand what DNA does wrong until we understand what it is responding to. And we have no promising hypotheses about the environmental contribution—no place to start looking. DNA is a chemical and it interacts with other chemicals; but our present concepts of environmental factors are at levels far too abstract to produce hypotheses at the chemical level. This will prove to be a major impediment to the development of wise and effective interventions in psychiatric disease. For example, "stress," as used in environmental studies, almost always lacks measurable physical properties, so it is undefined and untranslatable into chemicals that might interact with DNA. We shall have to translate "stress" to the levels described in Box 9 before its full meaning becomes available to us.

The study of schizophrenia is instructive. Perhaps more effort has gone into discovering the environmental factors that contribute to schizophrenia than into associating environmental factors with any other medical condition. Yet investigators cannot specify a single environmental contributor to the development of schizophrenia. At the present time, given a newborn infant known to have DNA compatible with schizophrenia (determining this will soon be possible), we could neither caution against environmental conditions that would produce schizophrenia nor specify any that would prevent it. Not a different mother, not gentler toilet training, not freedom from poverty, not avoiding preservatives in bread, not curtailing acid rain—no prescription based on evidence could be offered to help prevent schizophrenia. Indeed, any adjustment of environment that today might be devised in order to prevent the development of schizophrenia would probably have no effect, and if it did have an effect, it would be as likely to hurt as to help. A basic test of science—accurate prediction of the effects of actions taken—is thereby failed. The same is true of affective illness, the anxiety states, and so on through most psychiatric diseases. One exception is chemical dependence. Here we can specify environmental factors, such as alcohol. Without alcohol, there is no alcoholism.

There are two main reasons why we know so little about the contribution of environment to psychiatric illness. First, for both ethical and practical reasons, the skull has blocked experimental access to the brain. Human brain science has suffered as a result. In fact, much of what was known about the human brain a decade ago was actually discovered through chance opportunities to bypass the skull. Neurosurgical operations on the brain were one source of information. Disease, such as stroke, was another, because behavioral lapses recorded during life could be correlated with brain damage observed at autopsy. But these crude methods were scientifically unsatisfying as a basis for the study of disease.

Human brain science has also lagged behind because animal experimentation is of limited utility with respect to brain research on human diseases. Because animal proteins are not much different from our own, animal research has contributed enormously to our knowledge of cellular machinery and of small molecules such as neurotransmitters. It has also contributed to our grasp of the basic elements of behavior demonstrated by operant and Pavlovian conditioning, which have been and will continue to be indispensable tools for brain research. But our understanding of how complex, uniquely human reactions to environment are accomplished has not been greatly enhanced by animal research.

Although humans and certain animals are similar enough in liver, heart, and kidney to permit reasonably direct transfer of experimental results, this is not true of the brain. Humans use far more of their genetic material than any other animal (about 70 percent) exclusively for brain function. Animals exhibit the general range of human diseases, but they exhibit few of our brain diseases. It is not just that we cannot recognize a disease such as depression in an animal. Animal brains simply do not develop the same pathology as human brains—not the profusion of plaques and tangles seen in Alzheimer's disease, not the atrophy of Huntington's disease, not changes seen in other human brain diseases. Nothing will substitute for observations of the actual living human brain doing its routine work and responding to experimental manipulations of its environment.

Happily, it is becoming possible to perform such manipulations in non-invasive ways. New methods of studying the brain via imaging techniques have been developed. These techniques enable scientists to examine accurate representations of living brains and, in more advanced application, to compare ill brains directly to healthy ones as they respond to specific challenges. The first of these techniques to emerge was *computerized axial tomography*. The CAT scan takes static x-ray pictures of the brain, but a computer is used to construct artificial "slices" of the brain at different levels. These slices make it possible to "see" anatomic detail inside the brain. The same artificial slicing techniques underlie the much more sophisticated imaging technologies known as *magnetic resonance imaging* (MRI), *positron emitting tomography* (PET), and *single-photon emission computed tomography* (SPECT). (Single-photon technology seems at this time to be especially promising. The equipment required is relatively inexpensive, which means that most research centers will be able to develop it.) These technologies can detect changes in selected areas of the brain with a resolution approaching a quarter of a centimeter. This means that the effects of environmental manipulations such as drugs, sensory stimulation, and activation of memories can be studied in living persons—ill or well, male or female, old or young—without risk of harm and with minimum inconvenience. These more sophisticated forms of imaging are today's research tools. It will be a while before we know how useful they will prove in general medical practice. But exhilaration is building within psychiatry, as at last we can see through the skull to study the living brain doing its work.

Psychiatric Practice

The new genetics that is taking psychiatry by storm brings with it critical issues for both medical practice and society. Being able to pinpoint on DNA segments vulnerability specific to diseases implies the ability to predict who is likely to become ill with which disease. At this time, the precision of the localization is exact enough to allow prediction only for Huntington's disease. But several other diseases will soon be as well known. The DNA segments associated with disease can then be identified soon after conception and used to predict the occurrence of disease decades later. In the case of Huntington's disease, the prediction is nearly 100 percent accurate, because all gene carriers eventually develop the disease. In the case of schizophrenia, the prediction will be about 50 percent accurate because twin studies demonstrate that about half of gene carriers develop the disease, and the risk will be more ambiguous because an additional proportion of relatives will develop schizoid disorders.

Most psychiatric diseases are more like schizophrenia than Huntington's disease in this respect. Of course, no matter what the disease, these predictions would be of tremendous value to individuals if only we knew how to prevent the illness from developing—if only we knew what the environmental triggers are and how to adjust them. In all likelihood, however, we will have the power to identify disease carriers long before we learn how diseases can be prevented. Indeed, it now seems certain that any environmental manipulations we could devise, no matter how soundly based in theory, would have to be tested over the course of a generation, because the people at risk would have to live long enough to either develop or escape the disease. Meanwhile, policies need to be established to apply during a period when we can predict outcome but have no way to influence it.

This is in fact the situation faced today by persons with Huntington's disease. People carrying the DNA needed for the disease can be identified anytime after conception, although the disease is rarely manifest before middle age. (An average of 50 percent of the children of a parent who has the disease inherit the faulty DNA.) The disease is devastating: 12 to 15 years of progressive physical and mental deterioration lead to death. There is no effective treatment. When the faulty DNA is present, the eventual development of disease is certain; when it is not present, there is no risk.

When DNA testing is offered, what is the response of those at risk, most of whom have seen a parent sicken and die from the disease and therefore know what to expect? Some simply don't want to know whether they well get the disease or not and so decline the test. Others do want to know; if they then go through with the testing, they get either very good or very bad news. Those who find that they do not have Huntington's DNA describe themselves as ecstatic even if they hadn't expected to be so moved. "The weight of the world came off my shoulders" is a common reaction. Most people accept bad news with unexpected calm. This is partly because the centers doing the counseling have prepared well in both performing the test and imparting the information. But the calm is deceptive. No matter how well prepared one is, the bad news is devastating and adjustment is painful. Some people are judged too unstable to receive the news should it be bad and are therefore told that they are ineligible for the testing. No one is happy about this paternalistic granting or refusal of screening, but no one knows a better way to manage the problem.

Who should have the information about an individual's genetic risk? It cannot be kept secret if it is to help people at risk. Treating physicians need the information. And if insurance companies pay for the medical care, surely they have a right to know what they are paying for. Of course, if insurance companies know, their coverage will eventually reflect that knowledge. Prohibiting such adjustments would force insurance rates higher for those not at risk for particular illnesses. Eventually, those whose DNA is compatible with long life would be paying for those less fortunate. The alternative seems equally unfair. Those with faulty DNA would not only become ill earlier in life but would also be forced to pay all the costs of their bad fortune. And the insurance dilemmas seem relatively minor! Should governments have the right to know which citizens are vulnerable to illness? Should industry? Should a person with DNA predisposing to Huntington's disease or bipolar illness or Alzheimer's disease be allowed to become an airline pilot, a physician, an admiral, or President?

Such questions will plague us until effective treatments, especially preventive ones, are developed. But after treatments are discovered, we will enter a world now hard to imagine. In principle, nearly all psychiatric disease could then be prevented—and at little cost. Alzheimer's disease provides a typical example. In identical twins who develop Alzheimer's disease, the average difference in age at onset is 10 years. One twin develops this devastating disease, but the other remains completely well for an average of an additional 10 years. Indeed, some such co-twins never develop the disease.

I have been personally following one such identical pair. These women are now age 62. One of them developed Alzheimer's disease 11 years ago and is now bedfast, unable even to recognize her twin. The other twin remains perfectly well. She is examined every 6 months with the full battery of diagnostic tests, but so far there is not a hint of intellectual decline. Despite my mildly stated cautions, she is overweight, smokes a pack a day, and admits to taking at least one glass of wine each evening. She has DNA predisposing to Alzheimer's disease, but she remains perfectly well. Moreover, she does not take any medicine or suffer any of the other medical intrusions on normal life that are sometimes needed to keep disease in check.

The discordance in these identical twins must be attributed to post-conception events. Once we understand the rules of environmental interaction with DNA that have resulted in at least an added 11 years of healthy life, we should be able to double that to 22 years, and double it again to 44, and so on. And we should be able to apply that understanding in an effort to prevent the disease from developing at all. The same logic applies to nearly all psychiatric illness. That is the promise of the new psychiatry to psychiatric patients and their families.

Appendix A

Suggestions for Further Reading

□ □ □

THIS book is intended to bring highly technical material to a general audience that would not find technical sources useful. However, the following largely non-technical publications should provide greater depth and different perspectives for those who wish to read further on specific topics.

Chapter 1

Dalton, K. *Depression after Childbirth: How to Recognize and Treat Postnatal Illness*, 2nd ed. New York: Oxford University Press, 1989.

Hirschfield, R. A. *Depression: What We Know.* Available from Science Communications Branch, NIMH, Room 15C-17, 5600 Fishers Lane, Rockville, MD 20857.

Robins, E. *The Final Months: A Study of the Lives of 134 Persons Who Committed Suicide*. New York: Oxford University Press, 1981.

Roth, M., and J. Kroll. *The Reality of Mental Illness*. Cambridge, England: Cambridge University Press, 1986.

Storr, A. *Churchill's Black Dog, Kafka's Mice, and Other Phenomena of the Human Mind*. New York: Grove Press, 1988.

Useful Information on Suicide. Department of Health and Human Services, Washington, DC. DHHS Publication No. (ADM) 86-1489, 1986. Available from Science Communications Branch, NIMH, Room 15C-17, 5600 Fishers Lane, Rockville, MD 20857.

Chapter 2

Fieve, R. R. Moodswing, *The Third Revolution in Psychiatry*. New York: Morrow, 1975. A classic popularization dealing with affective illness. Accurate, authorative.

Hershman, D. J., and J. Lieb. *The Key to Genius: Manic-Depression and the Creative Life*. Buffalo, NY: Prometheus Books, 1988.

Livermore, J. M., C. P. Malmquist, and P. E. Meehl. "On the Justification for Civil Commitment." *The University of Pennsylvania Law Review* 117 (1968):75–96. A thoughtful article on the bases for judicial commitment.

Ellis, A. *Reason and Emotion in Psychotherapy*. New York: Lyle Stuart, 1963. Still an authoritative and readable source.

Jefferson, J. and J. Greist. *Primer of Lithium Therapy*. Baltimore, MD: Williams & Wilkins, 1977. Technical in parts but still readable.

Sloan, R. B., et al. *Psychotherapy Versus Behavior Therapy.* Cambridge, MA: Harvard University Press, 1975. Still the best study of treatment efficacy.

Chapter 3

Atkinson, J. M. *Schizophrenia at Home: A Guide to Helping the Family.* London, England: Croom Helm, 1986.

Gottesman, I. I., and J. Shields. *Schizophrenia and Genetics: A Twin Study Vantage Point.* New York: Academic Press, 1972. Surveys the genetic evidence demonstrating the contribution of genetics to schizophrenia. Also an informative introduction to the uses of twins in research.

Gottesman, I. I. *Schizophrenia Genesis: The Origins of Madness.* New York: W. H. Freeman, 1991. The best and most up-to-date general introduction.

Neals, J. M., and T. F. Oltmanns. *Schizophrenia.* New York: Wiley, 1980. College-level psychology.

"Residential Care and Treatment of the Chronic Mental Patient," *Psychiatric Annals*, vol. 15, no. 11, M. Blaustein, guest editor. Several generally readable, mostly non-technical articles on the problems posed by the chronic patient and possible approaches to them.

Torrey, E.F. *Nowhere to Go: The Tragic Odyssey of the Homeless Mentally Ill.* Harper & Row. New York, 1988.

Torrey, E. F. *Surviving Schizophrenia: A Family Manual (Revised).* New York: Harper & Row, 1988.

Chapter 4

Heston, L. L., and J. A. White. *The Vanishing Mind: A Practical Guide to Alzheimer's Disease and Other Dementias.* New York: W. H. Freeman, 1991.

Mace, N. L., and P. V. Rabins. *The 36-hour Day: A Family Guide to Caring for Persons with Alzheimer's Disease, Related Dementing Illnesses, and Memory Loss in Later Life.* Baltimore, MD: Johns Hopkins University Press, 1981.

Oliver, R. *Coping with Alzheimer's: A Caregiver's Emotional Survival Guide.* New York: Dodd, Mead, 1987.

Safford, F. *Caring for the Mentally Impaired Elderly: A Family Guide.* New York: Holt, 1986.

Psychiatric Treatment of Alzheimer's Disease. Committee on Aging, Group for the Advancement of Psychiatry. Available from Brunner/Mazel Publishers, 19 Union Square, New York, NY 10003.

Chapter 5

Eysenck, H. J., and S. Rachman. *The Causes and Cures of Neurosis: An Introduction to Modern Behavior Therapy Based on Learning Theory and the Principles of Conditioning.* San Diego, CA: R. R. Knapp, 1965. A classic that launched the conditioning therapies. Still provocative, still applicable.

DuPont, R. L., ed. *Phobia: A Comprehensive Summary of Modern Treatments.* New York: Brunner/Mazel, 1982. Uneven quality of articles, but most are quite good.

Rapoport, J. L., ed. *Obsessive-Compulsive Disorder in Children and Adolescents.* Washington DC: American Psychiatric Press, 1989. Comprehensive, current.

Reed, G. F. *Obsessional Experience and Compulsive Behavior: A Cognitive-Structural Appproach.* New York: Academic Press, 1985.

Turner, S. R., and D. C. Beidel. *Treating Obsessive-Compulsive Disorder.* New York: Pergamon Press, 1988. A knowledgeable survey of modern psychological methods.

Chapter 6

Fillmore, K. M. *Alcohol Use Across the Life Course: A Critical Review of 70 Years of International Longitudinal Research.* Toronto, Canada: Addiction Research Foundation, 1988. Comprehensive, detailed.

Johnson. V. E. *I'll Quit Tomorrow.* New York: Harper & Row, 1973. A moving first-person account of alcoholism.

Chapter 7

Bethune, H. *Off the Hook: Coping with Addiction.* London, England: Methuen, 1985.

Dorn, N. *Helping Drug Users.* Brookfield, VT: Gower, 1985.

Robins, L. N. *The Vietnam Drug User Returns.* Special Action Office Monograph, Series A, No. 2. Washington, DC: Special Action Office for Drug Abuse Prevention, Executive Office of the President, 1974.

Shah, N. S., and A. G. Donald (eds). *Endorphins and Opiate Antagonists in Psychiatric Research: Clinical Implications.* New York: Plenum Medical Book Co., 1982.

Chapter 8

Reid, W. H., ed. *Unmasking the Psychopath: Antisocial Personality and Related Syndromes*. New York: W. W. Norton, 1986.

Robins, L. N. *Deviant Children Grown Up: A Sociological and Psychiatric Study of Sociopathic Personality*. Baltimore, MD: Williams & Wilkins, 1966. The standard work in the field.

Smith, R. J. *The Psychopath in Society*. New York: Academic Press, 1978.

Chapter 9

Ackroyd, P. *Dressing Up: Transvestism and Drag*. New York: Simon & Schuster, 1979. A popular account. Overdone in places but a sympathetic, readable description.

Bayer, R. *Homosexuality and American Psychiatry. The Politics of Diagnosis, with a New Afterward About AIDS and Homosexuality*. Princeton, NJ: Princetion University Press, 1988. Strong sociopolitical slant, a definite viewpoint.

Hare, E. H. "The Origin and spread of Dementia Paralytica." *Journal of Mental Science* 105 (1959):594-626. A scholarly account of the syphilitic brain disease epidemic. Comprehensive references. (The *Journal of Mental Science* is now known as *The British Journal of Psychiatry*.)

Jones, D. P. H., and M. G. McQuiston. *Interviewing the Sexually Abused Child*. London, England: Royal College of Psychiatrists, 1977.

Shilts, R. *And the Band Played On: Politics, People, and the AIDS Epidemic*. New York: St. Martin's, 1987. A excellent popularized account.

Turner, C. F., H. G. Milller, and L. E. Moses. eds. *AIDS: Sexual Behavior and Intravenous Drug Use*. Washington, DC: National Academy Press, 1989. A National Research Council review of the problem. Comprehensive. Technical in places, but most of the book easily understandable.

Chapter 10

Andreasen, N. C., ed. *Brain Imaging in Psychiatry*. Washington, DC: American Psychiatric Press, 1988. Technical, but most articles are understandable.

Kinzey, W. G. ed. *The Evolution of Human Behavior:Primate Models*. New York: SUNY Press, 1986.

Monad, J. *Chance and Necessity: An Essay on the Natural Philosophy of Modern Biology*. Translated by A. Wainhouse. New York: Vintage Books, 1972. A profound essay on mutation and evolution.

The Molecules of Life. New York: W. H. Freeman, 1985. Readings from *Scientific American*.

Mapping and Sequencing the Human Genome. Report of the Committee on Mapping and Sequencing the Human Genome. Available from National Academy Press, 2101 Constitution Avenue, N.W., Washington, DC.

Tanner, N. *On Becoming Human*. Cambridge, England: Cambridge University Press, 1981.

Vanderberg, S. G., S. M. Singer., and D. L. Pauls. *The Heredity of Behavior Disorders in Adults and Children*. New York: Plenum, 1985.

The Neuroscience of Mental Health: A Report on Neuroscience Research. Available from U.S. Department of Health and Human Services, Alcohol, Drug Abuse, and Mental Health Administration, Rockville, MD 20857. A comprehensive review of neurobiology relevant to illness. Requires some background in biology.

Appendix B

Support Groups and Other Sources of Help

□ □ □

ONE OF the very promising developments of the past decade has been the rise of support groups. Most of these organizations have chapters in all major population centers and so are within reach of most ill persons and their families. They provide information not only through more formal channels, such as publications and sponsored meetings, but also through personal exchanges with ordinary people who have had first-hand experience with an illness. Such support groups are also, increasingly, acting as advocates for the ill, bringing their special problems to the attention of political organizations and the public at large. The names, addresses, and telephone numbers of some of these groups follow.

AIDS Referral
1620 Eye St., N.W.
Washington, DC 20006
202-293-7330

Al-Anon Family Group Headquarters
1372 Broadway
New York, NY 10018
212-302-7240
(For families affected by alcoholism)

Alcoholics Anonymous
P.O. Box 459
Grand Central Station
New York, NY 10163
212-686-1100

For a catalogue of federal publications on alcohol and drug abuse,
write to:
National Clearinghouse for Alcohol and Drug Abuse Information
P.O. Box 2345
Rockville, MD 20857

Alzheimer's Disease and Related Diseases Association
919 N. Michigan Avenue,
Chicago, Il 60611
800-621-0379
(One of the most valuable to affected families)

American Association of Suicidology
2458 South Ash
Denver, CO 80222
(Primarily a support organization)

Depression After Delivery
P.O. Box 1282
Morrisville, PA 19607
(Information and support for those affected by post partum depression)

Drug Abuse
Cocaine Anonymous
Narcotics Anonymous
P.O. Box 9999
Van Nuys, CA 97409
818-989-7841
(Modeled on Alcoholics Anonymous).

The federal agency charged with research and education in drug abuse, excepting alcohol, maintains a hotline number National Institute of Drug Abuse, 800-622-4357. Spanish-language callers may use 800-662-9832.

National Alliance of Mental Patients
P.O. Box 618
Souix Falls, SD 57101
605-334-4067

The National Alliance for the Mentally Ill
1901 North Fort Myer Drive
Suite 500
Arlington, VA 22209
703-524-7600
(One of the most effective of all advocacy groups)

National Depressive and Manic Depressive Association
Merchandise Mart
P.O Box 3395
Chicago, IL 60654
312-993-0066

National Foundation for Depressive Illness, Inc.
20 Charles St.
New York, NY 10014
800-248-4344

National Mental Health Association
1021 Prince St.
Alexandria, VA 22314
703-684-7722

Neurotics Anonymous
PO Box 4866
Cleveland Park Station
Washington, DC 20006
202-628-4379

OCD Foundation, Inc.
P.O. Box 9573
New Haven, CT 06535
203-772-0665
(Support and information for those affected by obsessional illness.)

Phobia Society of America
133 Rollins Ave.
Suite 4B
Rockville, MD 20853
301-231-9350

Recovery, Inc.
802 North Dearborn St.
Chicago, IL 60610
312-337-5661
(Mainly a support group for discharged patients)

Schizophrenia Association of America
900 N. Federal Highway
Suite 330
Boca Raton, FL 33432
800-847-3802

Index

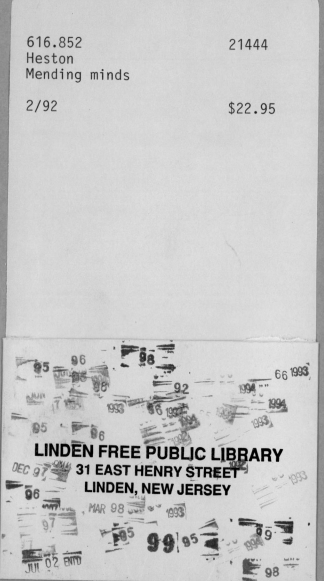